I0413830

A WORLD
WITHOUT
SMELLS

LARS LUNDQVIST

2017

Copyright © 2017 Lars Lundqvist

All rights reserved.

ISBN: 1542840104
ISBN-13: 978-1542840101

Cover photo: My Good Images/Shutterstock.com

To Elsy,
for teaching me
about smells

CONTENTS

Prologue—For Those Who Can Smell

IF YOU HAD to give up one of your senses, which would you choose? Sight? Hearing? Touch? Not very likely. So if the choice stands between smell and taste, what would you choose? Most people probably choose the sense of smell, possibly thinking that they would not want to be without the taste of food and that smells are not that important in a modern society. But do they really understand what they would miss without a sense of smell?

The sense of smell is somewhat like an undercover sense. You seldom notice it, but it is continuously working, informing you about your surroundings. Often you do not even think about it. Imagine a summer morning. You are lying in your bed, eyes closed, listening to the morning sounds. Through the half-open window you suddenly hear an engine working somewhere and at first you cannot identify what it is, but then you realize that it probably is the neighbor who is mowing his lawn. You hardly noticed the whiff of freshly cut grass but it was enough to let your brain draw the correct conclusion. Next, you smell coffee and realize that someone has already begun making breakfast.

Lars Lundqvist

Even before you open your eyes, your sense of smell has given you information about your surroundings, and not only about what is happening in your bedroom, but also about things occurring elsewhere, like the neighbor mowing his lawn and somebody making coffee in the kitchen. Smells tell you that someone is baking bread, that spring is in the air, that it is time to change the baby's diaper, that bread in the toaster is getting burnt, that your neighbor has lit his grill, that dinner is on the stove. The sense of smell can carry information from far away, about things that are beyond hearing or sight. And most of all, what you perceive as taste is actually mostly smell.

But what if there were no smells? Imagine that summer morning again, lying in your bed. You hear the engine working but there are no smells to help you identify what it is. You have to get up and look out the window to see the neighbor mowing his lawn. And there is nothing to inform you that someone has started the coffee machine, until you go down to the kitchen and see it.

Try to imagine the world you know, with all its familiar things, but without smells. If you have ever had a really bad cold you probably know what it feels like when your sense of smell does not work properly. That gives you an indication what it would be like to lose your sense of smell. But what if smells had never existed? How would that have changed your perception of the world, and how would it change your everyday life?

For a small group of people that is the way the world is. I am one of those. I was born without a sense of smell, so to me smells do not exist and never have. I live my life in the midst of your world, without you noticing that my smell-free world is very different from your smell-centered world. And sometimes our worlds collide, especially when I have to adapt myself and my life to all your rules about smells.

Prologue—for those who can smell

In this book I will try to describe my world without smells, and what it is like to live in a world where everyone else perceives a dimension that does not exist in my world.

PART ONE

I am anosmic!

I am alone!

LET US START from the beginning.

Anosmia.

Have you heard the word before? Probably not. Anosmia comes from the Greek words *an* meaning "without" and *osme* meaning "smell". Together they mean "not having a sense of smell". Everyone knows that blind means that you cannot see, and deaf that you cannot hear, but there is no simple word for "not sensing smells". Not even those who are anosmic usually know that their condition is called anosmia and neither did I.

Anosmia is an invisible condition. You quickly notice if someone is blind or deaf, but how do you notice if someone is anosmic? It does not show on the outside, or in the way we anosmics behave. An anosmic communicates in the same way that everybody else does, eats the same food, and appears to function just like anyone else.

There are two kinds of anosmia; acquired, which means that you lose your sense of smell at some point in life, and congenital, which means that you are born without the sense.

I am a congenital anosmic so I have lived my whole life without a sense of smell. To me it is natural that there are no smells. It has always been like that. My world has always been without smells and I usually do not think at all about smells.

So what was it that triggered me to start looking for information about anosmia at the age of 57 and made me write this book? Strange as it may seem it was the absence of a comment.

Everything started with my wife going away over the weekend to visit a relative while I stayed at home taking care of our horses, cats and the dog. On Saturday afternoon, around five, I was sitting with my laptop doing something, when it suddenly occurred to me that it was like a normal weekday when I was working from home, except for one aspect. My wife would not come home from work and say something about stuffy air or some bad smell in our house. Good!

What? Where did that "Good!" come from?

My reaction surprised me, to say the least. I had never thought that comments about smells had bothered me, but my own reaction made me realize that they obviously did, in a way that I had never really understood. So I began to analyze things that had happened in the past, things that had been said over the years, and how I had handled different situations involving smells. And I suddenly realized that although my wife, my children, my siblings, my parents, everyone close to me, rationally know that I have no sense of smell, they do not know what that actually means. They do not understand the ultimate consequence of living in a world without smells and how I really do not understand anything about smells. But what really shocked me was when I realized that I myself had never really understood this either.

It all ended with me sitting on the floor, crying. It was partly because I finally admitted to myself that I really did not understand anything about this thing called smell, but perhaps even more because I realized that no one else could understand how it felt to be so totally cut off from a whole dimension of the world that everyone else was experiencing. And most of all, the feeling of being completely alone about this. How could others

I am alone!

understand anything about something I hardly understood myself?

I had been living with this for 57 years, and had always joked about it, pointing out the advantages of not having to smell anything bad. I had never really admitted, not even to myself, that there were problems as well, disadvantages, and that absence of a sense of smell is a disability.

When I had finished crying, it occurred to me that there must be others without a sense of smell. I could hardly be unique. There should be information somewhere. So I started to search the internet.

I AM NOT ALONE!

MY FIRST SURPRISE was that my condition had a name: anosmia. The second surprise was that there was almost no information in Swedish on congenital anosmia. I thought that books about the topic should exist, or official information on the internet, but I found almost nothing in Swedish. There were a few articles about anosmia in some local newspapers, but usually about acquired anosmia, about people who lost their sense of smell as an adult. In the very few articles about congenital anosmia it was usually presented as a funny curiosity, and never taken seriously.

So I wrote to the National Board of Health and Welfare (Socialstyrelsen), the government agency in Sweden that falls under the Ministry of Health and Social Affairs. Its responsibility is to "ensure good health, social welfare and high-quality health and social care on equal terms for the whole Swedish population". I asked for information about "isolated congenital anosmia," which means that you are born without a sense of smell but otherwise healthy. The answer from their "Information center for Rare Diseases" was that "We have no separate information on isolated anosmia". Next, I wrote to the "Swedish Disability Federation," the umbrella organization in which 39 disability organizations co-operate to be the "united voice of the Swedish disability movement before government, the parliament and national authorities". I thought that maybe they would have some information on anosmia? The answer I got was "Have you tried the National Board of Health and Welfare?"

Congenital anosmia obviously does not exist in official Sweden. One might wonder why.

When I could not find any relevant information in Swedish, I began searching for information in English instead, and suddenly I found a whole new world. There were all sorts of web pages on anosmia, and many blogs. Some active, some inactive. I found associations, mailing lists, and finally the Facebook group "Congenital anosmia".

I can still remember the initial feeling when I joined the group. It was the first time I got in touch with other congenital anosmics:

"Wow! Others like me! Finally! People who understand what it is like to be anosmic!"

And above all, "I am not alone!"

The discussions in this group really has helped me in my attempts to understand my own anosmia. I found answers to my questions, tips on web pages and articles on congenital anosmia, and could compare my experiences with those of others.

Suddenly I had somewhere to share my thoughts about anosmia. A place where my experiences were not seen as unusual or abnormal, but quite normal and ordinary. I read what others had posted, read their comments, asked questions, commented on others' posts, and so on. The feeling of relief was enormous. I was in a state of euphoria for several days.

While searching the internet for information on anosmia I made a list of problems, advantages and disadvantages in my everyday life. I read about the sense of taste, tried to learn about the sense of smell and different kinds of problems that could occur. After a while I decided to organize all the information in a more systematic way. The end result was this book. It became a

I am not alone!

way for me to understand and accept my own anosmia, and to come to terms with the realization that I have lived my whole life in a world without smells.

What is it like to live with anosmia from birth? How does it affect my day-to-day life? The easiest way to describe it is to tell you about an ordinary day, and to show you when I am reminded of or affected by my anosmia.

AN ORDINARY DAY

IT IS A normal day in mid May. The snow melted early this year, so the grass is already green, but the buds of the birches are still sleeping. Spring flowers have just emerged in the flowerbed beside the porch. The alarm clock wakes me up just after 6 AM as usual. When I enter the kitchen my wife mentions that we forgot to take the garbage outside the previous evening, so there was an unpleasant smell in the kitchen when she came down. I answer "Okay" and drop the garbage in the dustbin outside, when on my way to pick up the morning newspaper. On my way to the postbox I notice that the grass and the driveway looks wet. It seems it rained during the night. When I am back in the kitchen I serve myself a bowl of cereal with milk, but notice that the Best-before date of the milk expired yesterday, so I ask my wife to smell it, to check that it is okay. After a quick breakfast I go upstairs to take a shower, and get a comment in the passing from my wife, telling me to change my towel. The one I have been using does not smell very nice, so I toss it in the laundry basket and pick a new one.

Driving into town we listen to a local radio station, and I think about the work to be done during the day, when my wife suddenly says that she smells something burning. I wonder if it has to do with the car, but as we keep driving the smell disappears, so my wife guesses that we passed a farm where they were burning something.

At work we have morning coffee around 9 AM. A co-worker mentions a smelly lunch box left in the sink since yesterday. I didn't notice, of course, but my colleagues make faces and say it's disgusting.

For lunch I brought leftovers from Sunday dinner. Standing at the microwave oven a colleague comments about someone having had salmon for lunch, and how heating it in the microwave makes the whole lunch room stink. What? How can nice food stink? To avoid a complicated discussion I ignore the comment.

In the afternoon, when we gather for a coffee break, someone asks about a weird smell in the corridor outside the labs. Another colleague explains what it is, emphasizing that it is harmless.

After work and coming home, my wife says "Leave the door open, it feels stuffy". When I answer "What?" she says "It smells".

After dinner it is time to go down to the stables to take care of our horses. The stable doors are wide open although it is chilly outside. One of the other horse owners says she left the doors open because of a thick smell of urine. My wife also comments on it and asks me if I really can't feel it. But no, I don't sense anything unusual in the stables. The air is the same as always, the same as outside the stables, or out in the yard, or in our house, or at work. Air can have different temperatures, and different humidity, but apart from that air is always just air.

We take the horses inside, groom them, and ride a tour around the village. My wife says there is a smell of smoke, and after a while I see a small column of smoke. One of the villagers is burning last year's grass and twigs. We eventually return to the stables and leave the horses indoors for the night.

Returning to the house I leave my boots outside because I

know my wife wants me to. From what I have heard they smell strongly when coming directly from the stables.

Just before bedtime I remember I worked up a sweat while riding and taking care of the horses, so I take a shower before going to bed.

My ordinary anosmic day is over.

ANALYZING THE DAY

THE MAIN DIFFERENCE between us, congenital anosmics, and persons with a functioning sense of smell probably is that we never spontaneously think about smells, except as an abstract phenomenon when someone comments on it. I do not wake up in the morning thinking "Wow, I still can't smell anything". When I wake up, I think about anything except smells.

This particular day there had been twelve comments that made me think about smells. They were about the garbage in the kitchen, the milk, my towel, a smell of something burnt while driving to town, the smelly lunch box, someone heating salmon in the microwave, a smell in the corridor, bad air in our house, smell of urine in the stables, smoke in the village, boots on the porch, having worked up a sweat.

How often I think about smells on any given day depends on my surroundings. If no one says anything about smells during the day, I usually do not think about it at all. Twelve times, like on this particular day, is probably more than average. Then there are days when it is mentioned all the time, especially during spring and summer, when there appear to be smells everywhere. But comments about flowers and other things that smell nice often pass me by unnoticed. It is only when I have to react to the comments that I really notice them, and that usually means bad smells. Others sensing nice smells does not really matter to me.

Maybe you noticed that "using deodorant" was not in the list.

Does that mean I do not use deodorant? No, I do use a deodorant, but doing that is part of my morning ritual. Strange as it may seem, this is not something that I immediately associate with smells, because to me the deodorant does not have a smell. Nor is "using clean clothes" on the list, for the same reason. As a kid I was taught that I have to change clothes, so when I put yesterdays t-shirt in the laundry bin I just follow routine. It is not because it smells of sweat because I actually do not know if it does. I do it because it is what you do. You wash clothes that have been used.

Neither "spring flowers" nor "wet grass and driveway" were on the list of things that reminded me of smells, for the simple reason that I was alone. No one mentioned how the flowers or the grass smelled. I saw the flowers and the wet grass, but I do not associate either flowers, rain or grass with smells.

In the end it is very simple. If someone mentions smells, especially bad smells, I notice and think about it. If no one does, I seldom think about smells or my anosmia. And even when I think about smells, I do not think about the smells themselves. I think about the abstract phenomenon 'smell'. The milk in the morning is a good example. When I noticed that the Best-before date had expired and asked my wife to smell it, I did it so she could decide if I could use it, not because I wanted to know what the exact smell was.

When I started writing this chapter, my original plan was to have my wife describe the same day from the perspective of someone who can smell, to list all the instances she noticed smells, and then to compare her and my list. It sounded like a good idea, from my perspective. What I forgot was that a person who can smell senses smells all the time, and usually without consciously thinking about it. It would be like asking a seeing person to keep a list of all the moments when she thinks about using her sense of sight and comparing that with a list of occasions when a blind person is reminded of her blindness. I am sometimes reminded about not having a sense of smell, but a person who has always had that sense is never reminded about having it, because it has always been there. We are literally living in two different worlds and they cannot be described in the same way.

But how did my anosmic life begin?

GROWING UP WITH ANOSMIA

WHEN I LOOK back at my early childhood, I have no memories of thinking about smells. I do not remember wondering what smell was, or thinking I was missing out on something. I do not even remember people talking about smells in my day-to-day life. I assume that my parents and other adults mentioned smells every now and then, like they did when I got older, but the only thing I remember is that I early on saw it as a kind of game, something people just said. When someone audibly farted, everyone else protested, vigorously displaying disgust, and so did I! I thought it was the sound everyone else was reacting to, so I mimicked their behavior, not understanding that there was more than sound involved.

When my parents read me books with stories and fairy tales, smells were sometimes mentioned, but also magic, gnomes, trolls, and other things that do not exist. In the animated movies I loved to watch, animals often sniffed at things, or tracked something, the way I had seen real cats and dogs do. I think I just accepted the fact that animals could smell things, but human comments on smells were only a part of the play, a fantasy, not about something that really existed.

So I just tagged along and said the same things although I did not know what they meant. I do not remember exactly when I realized there was something I did not understand when my family and friends were talking about farts and stenches, or the scent of flowers, but I was probably about 10-11 years old when I finally understood that there actually was such a thing as smells, and that others could sense them, like when dogs sniffed things. Still, not being able to smell did not seem to affect my life in any way. Smells seemed unimportant, especially as no one noticed my inability to smell. However, I do remember two occasions when the grown-ups possibly should have reacted and wondered if something was different.

The first occasion was an ordinary afternoon when I was seven or eight years old. I was outside playing with my best friend at the time, the girl next door, when her mother suddenly called her in to have dinner. I waited outside until she had finished so we could continue playing. We kept playing for another hour or so, and then finally said, "Bye" and parted. When I got home my mother was angry because I had once more forgotten to come inside to have dinner. She was tired of always having to remind me of eating. Did I not get hungry? Did I not think about dinner when my friend went inside to eat? Did I not smell dinner? My answers to all those questions were "No". To teach me not to miss dinner again she would not heat the food again, so I would have to eat it cold. I remember thinking that this seemed fair and it really did not matter. After all, the food tasted roughly the same irrespective of being warm or cold. I do remember that my mother was a bit surprised that I ate the cold food with the same appetite as if it had been warm.

The second occasion happened during a summer holiday at my grandparents' farm in northern Sweden. One day all the adults were about to eat "surströmming," fermented herring, a traditional dish in northern Sweden. The fish has a very salty and somewhat acid taste, but most of all it smells a lot. A lot! Most people find the smell appalling, to say the least. Many even claim that it stinks, smells revolting, like rotten fish, and so on. From what I have heard, children usually react stronger to the smell than adults do, and sure enough all the children fled outdoors, except me. I stayed inside with the adults eating the fish, and I loved it. I remember the grown-ups asking me if I did not think that it smelled horrible, and that I truthfully answered "No". Looking back I wonder why no one reacted enough to repeat the question and tried to understand why my reaction was so different compared to the other children.

Thinking back I remember not understanding at all what they were talking about. At the time I was still too young to understand that the others had a sense which I did not have.

When I was eleven my family moved. This meant new school and new friends. By then I think I knew that there was something called smell, which others could sense. But I do not remember thinking about it and definitely not understanding it. Others mentioned it every now and then but as it did not exist to me it did not matter, so why bother?

I got a new best friend, a boy living in the house next to ours. We played every day, all kinds of games. We were mostly outdoors, playing soccer or street hockey, or playing various games in the nearby forest, but we also played a lot in my room. Afterwards, when he had gone home, my mother would enter the room and open the window, politely telling me that it sometimes smelled of "young boys" and that she actually preferred that we did not spend that much time indoors. I remember not understanding at all, especially as the way she said it suggested that it was mainly my friend who was responsible for the smell. After all, I slept in there and that never was reason to open the window.

Another memory is when I was in my early teens and my mother suggested that I should start using deodorant. As far as I remember I only said "Okay" because I already knew from commercials that people used it, so I simply accepted that I too had to do that. I do not remember thinking about why I should do it. I think I just saw it as another one of those incomprehensible things that grown-ups did and which was part of growing up.

I gradually learned that I could not smell, but not knowing what it meant, I did not think about it. I guess my mind was on set other things, things that existed and mattered. It took another few years before I understood that my parents did not know that I was anosmic. So one day I told them.

I AM ANOSMIC

AS A CHILD you assume your parents are all-knowing, so it was not until I was in my early teens that I broached the subject. They were surprised, to put it mildly, and hardly believed me. When I persisted they claimed it must have happened recently. Surely they would have noticed if their son did not react to smells? Looking back it is not at all strange that they never noticed anything. Anosmia was completely unknown back then. It still is, not even talked about in children's health care.

My history is not unique. On the contrary! Almost all anosmics I have been in touch with tell a similar story. As a child you learn to play along in the social game when people are talking about smells, without understanding that to others it is not a game; it is for real. A typical example is when people talk about food. My sense of taste works just fine, so I have always been able to taste the food I eat, but as a child I did not understand that what I tasted was not the same as what everyone else did. Now I know that part of my food preferences are probably affected by my anosmia but there are large differences in food preferences between persons who can smell as well, so my food preferences were never a good indication of my anosmia.

A child cannot understand that others experience the world in another way. Especially not when parents and other grown-ups do not notice anything being different. You need to have reached a certain degree of maturity, a level of abstract thinking, to be able to understand how other humans function. On top of that, anosmia is not something that is talked about so most children probably do not even know that there is such a thing as anosmia.

Children learn early on that people can be deaf and blind, from fairy tales and children's books, but also from the way people talk. When someone in the family is searching for something and can not find it, in spite of it lying in front of them, a sibling or parent might say "Can't you see it's right in front of you, are you blind?" Or when someone asks a child a question and does not get an immediate answer, the question might be followed by the comment "Hello, can't you hear me, are you deaf?" Furthermore, both blind and deaf are used metaphorically. One can be blind to something, or deaf to criticism. But the sense of smell is never used that way when people talk, so neither the sense of smell nor anosmia is ever present when people talk about other things. Anosmia is an invisible and unknown disability, which no one ever talks about with children. So if parents or other adults do not notice anything, a child often has to reach an age of at least 8-10 years before she herself can understand that she is different.

Sometimes anosmics think that this thing called "smelling" is something you have to learn, you have to train yourself, just like learning to ride a bicycle. But when all your friends have already learned to smell you would seem a bit odd if you admitted still not having learned it. So the anosmic does not say anything, and keeps trying to learn it, until it one day becomes obvious that it does not work.

So what happened after I had told them of my anosmia? Well, nothing really. My mother suggested I should see a doctor. Perhaps there was just some simple adjustment that needed to be done, like removing polyps or something, and then I would get it back? I said no because I could not see the point. There was nothing to restore. Smells did not exist. How could a doctor change that? I do not think that my parents really understood that my anosmia was congenital, that I was born this way and that my "condition" was normal to me.

I have read and heard many stories about congenital anosmics who have seen doctors to find the cause of their anosmia. Sometimes a cause was found, but very often not. When a child was examined, it sometimes ended with the doctor questioning the anosmia, suggesting that the child was not trying hard enough, or just pretending, thereby confirming the child's thoughts that perhaps she was doing something wrong.

When I was nineteen I left home to study at the Royal College of Forestry. My days were filled with studies, parties, hunting and social life. By now I did know that I had no sense of smell but when people wanted my opinion about something related to smells I always avoided the subject by giving vague answers. On a few occasions I did mention not being able to smell but the only response was a few irrelevant questions (from my point of view) and five minutes later everyone had forgotten all about it and asked me about smells again. So I stopped telling anyone and in doing so also made my best to more or less forget all about it myself. As far as I know no one of my class mates knew back then and still do not know that I am anosmic.

Looking back, I went through three different phases. First, as a child, I did not know that there was such a thing as smells and a sense of smell, so I did not think about it. Then one day at around 10-11 years old I understood that others had a sense that I did not have, but I did not understand the consequences or how it mattered, so I still did not think about it. But when I went to live on my own I suddenly found myself in situations where I was supposed to comment on smells or answer questions about smells. Still not understanding my anosmia or knowing how to handle it I always gave evading answers and comments and tried not to think about smells as much as possible.

In retrospect I have to admit that my tactics were successful, in a way. They enabled me to live for very many years without really having to deal with my anosmia. But I sometimes wonder how it could be that no one noticed that I was anosmic. It cannot be that hard to spot, can it?

Is your child anosmic?

IT USUALLY TAKES many years for a child with congenital anosmia to understand that she is different, that she lacks a sense that everyone else has. Considering the highly developed children's health care we have in Sweden, where all children are repeatedly medically checked during their first few years, it is odd, to say the least, that anosmia is not detected at an early stage. The reason for this is that the olfactory system is never tested, and that no one asks the parents questions that could help them to discover it. Eyesight, hearing and the ability to move in a normal way are tested, but not smell and taste. It is as if smell and taste are not a part of a child's state of health, as if it is of no consequence if a child has a functioning sense of smell or not. If you know what to look for it is fairly easy to discover anosmia when a child is very young.

The most obvious sign that one's child is anosmic is an *indirect* signal: the absence of spontaneous comments about smells. Early on, an anosmic child learns to play the "smell game," to participate in the social game and to respond correctly to comments about smells. But a child without a sense of smell will never spontaneously comment about smells. Understandably, an anosmic child can never make the first comment about something that she smells.

A number of parents with anosmic children are members in the Facebook group. When asked what made them realize that their child was anosmic, this was the most common answer, the absence of spontaneous comments. The second most common answer was that they gave indeterminate or evasive answers to direct questions about smells.

One mother described how her daughter came home from school one day with an orange covered with cloves. She showed it to her mother, commenting how funny and pretty it looked. "Yes, and it smells wonderful, doesn't it?" her mother answered. "Yes, really fresh!" the girl responded. When the mother compared it with other nicely smelling things the daughter answered "Yes, they also smell fresh!" At this point the mother had begun to suspect that something was amiss. She asked her daughter if she ever noticed things that smelled bad, or if she could smell what mother had been cooking for dinner when she came home from school. The little girl looked completely surprised and baffled. She did not understand what her mother meant. How could anyone know what mother was preparing for dinner without having seen the food?

It doesn't even have to be verbal comments. Even very small children react to foul smells by making faces and with body language, and as soon as children can talk they start making remarks about smells. I noticed early on that my children reacted to smells, like sniffing the food, or making faces, sounds and remarks when something smelled really bad, and they did this almost before they were able to talk. But the reason I observed this at such an early age was probably because I knew a child can be anosmic. If that thought never occurs to you, you obviously do not pay attention to it. Because it is only a question of being observant, and drawing the right conclusion. I will give an example of how wrong the conclusions might be even though all the correct signals are present, because anosmia is not even considered as an option.

Is your child anosmic?

It was an evening when I was 11 or 12 years old. I was having a cup of tea and some toast while my parents took an evening stroll around the block. The TV was on in the living-room next to the kitchen. We had an old manual toaster where you had to check the bread and eject it when done. I had popped in two slices of bread when I heard something interesting on the TV. So I went into the living-room to watch, just briefly, while waiting for the toast. The TV was positioned so I had my back towards the kitchen. It must have been something really interesting on the TV because I stayed in the living-room longer than planned. When my parents approached the house they saw me through the big panorama windows, sitting on the floor in front of the TV, totally mesmerized, and above me thick black smoke spreading under the ceiling. They hurried into the house shouting at me to turn off the toaster. I ran into the kitchen, pulled the plug from the wall, noticing that there was a lot of smoke under the kitchen ceiling. The two slices of bread looked like glowing charcoal, so it was probably pure luck that they had not caught fire.

"Did you not notice the smell of smoke?" they asked, chocked. As far as I remember I simply answered "No," because that was the way it was. I remember that my parents were pretty angry about the way I had neglected the toaster but also surprised that I had not sensed the smell of smoke. During the discussion that followed, several alternative explanations for this were suggested, like I had been sitting on the floor while the smoke was under the ceiling, or that I had been so totally focused on the TV. But no one suggested the most obvious alternative: I had not smelled the smoke because I could not smell at all.

My story is not unique. Several anosmics have told me the same story, about slices of bread being transformed into charcoal or catching fire when they were forgotten in the toaster. And just like in my case, it never occurred to anybody that the explanation could be the absence of a sense of smell.

Besides the absence of spontaneous comments about smells, there is another obvious sign: the child's lack of reactions to remarks about smells made by others, especially about bad smells. Since the child does not know what you are referring to, she usually does not react to the remarks. After all, to the child it is just words without any substantial meaning. A typical example is when an adult and a child enter a room where there is a really strong smell. When the adult makes a remark about the smell, it comes as a total surprise to the child. A normal reaction from the adult is to ask "Don't you notice the smell?" If the child then answers "No" I would draw the conclusion that it is quite possible that the child actually could not sense smells, at all.

I have been asked that same question at several occasions, also as an adult: "Did you notice the smell..," and truthfully answered "No" but almost never received the natural follow-up question, "Maybe you can't smell at all?"

But if you think that your child is anosmic, what should you do?

How can you be sure?

IF YOU SUSPECT that your child is anosmic the easiest way to make sure is to simply ask the child, like the mother did in the example above when the daughter brought home a scented orange. The next step is to test it in some way.

The most usual test is to present various substances to the child and tell her to identify them. I think that it is extremely important that the adults conducting the test really understand that if the child is anosmic, she will not understand the purpose of the test. If the test is done as a blind test, with the child being blindfolded, an anosmic child will not even know that various smelly substances are presented to her, much less what they are. It is important that the test is not treated as a pass-fail test, and that the parents or other adults clearly state that it is okay not to sense the smells, to not even understand what is happening, in case the child is anosmic. To avoid confusion it is important to choose substances that have a clear smell, but at the same time do not emit fumes that trigger the receptors of the trigeminal nerve. Herbs, flowers and garlic are good substances, while ammonia, menthol, camphor and vinegar are unsuitable, as they trigger the trigeminal nerve.

Having concluded that one's child does not react at all to smells, and apparently does not have a sense of smell, what is the next step? Should you visit an ENT (ear-nose-throat) clinic to get it confirmed with modern technique? It may seem obvious, but it might not be that simple.

A reason not to see a doctor at an early age is that if the child is congenitally anosmic, nothing can be done about it. Congenital anosmia cannot be cured. At best, a visit to an ENT clinic will give the parents an explanation for the child's anosmia, but at worst it will make things even more confusing for the child. The general level of knowledge about congenital anosmia is usually so low, also among practicing medical doctors, that the probability that the parents and the child will get relevant answers and advice is extremely low. For that reason you might as well wait until the child herself one day starts asking why.

In my discussions with other anosmics and parents of anosmics, I often get the feeling that finding the reason for the anosmia is usually more important to parents than to the anosmic herself. At an age of 8-10 years, most anosmic children know that they lack an ability that everyone else seems to have, and for most of them this insight is quite uncomplicated. They have nothing else to compare it with, and most things in life just move on as usual, without anyone else noticing.

But there is one reason that supports the notion to visit a doctor. In rare cases, congenital anosmia is a symptom of a more serious affliction. One example is Kallmann's syndrome, which is a congenital lack of certain hormones, preventing normal development during puberty. If it is spotted in time, the child can be treated with hormones and get a normal sexual development. In this case the anosmia serves as a warning for something else, so for that reason it might be a good idea to visit a doctor when the child approaches puberty.

Even if you do not visit a doctor or ENT clinic, it is of course an advantage from the child's point of view if the parents know that their child is anosmic. If people around me had understood, early on, that I could not sense smells, they could have helped me understand the concept, and helped me to handle things I could not handle myself.

But what if it is the parent who is anosmic, not the child?

BEING AN ANOSMIC PARENT

PARENTHOOD IS ONE of those things that is often discussed in our Facebook group and which sometimes worries anosmics. More than once I have heard anosmics express concern when they are expecting their first child, worrying that being anosmic will create a problem. Looking back at when we were expecting our first child, I cannot remember myself having any similar worries. And when our first child was born, I cannot recall that I ever experienced my anosmia to be a problem.

A common issue of concern when you have a baby is, of course, to know when to change diaper. I suppose someone who can smell uses smell as one of the cues indicating that it is time to change diaper, but it is not the only cue. The facial expression of the child and the increased weight of the diaper, are two other signals. To be certain, even those that can smell often take a peek inside the diaper, and then there is the very certain method of sticking your finger inside to feel the surface. It might sound disgusting but it is not. The poo of a small child being fed on breast milk looks like custard and it has no smell. At least not to me. For once my anosmia actually was an advantage. I guess all parents who can smell would think that a diaper that is not smelling even when it is full would be a great product, at least when changing diapers. Well, to me it was always like that so changing diapers never bothered me in the least. But there came a time when being anosmic more or less saved the day, although I did not really think about it that way at the time.

When our children began spending their days in the communal daycare and met a lot of other kids, they were suddenly exposed to all kinds of germs. It was no wonder that they became sick from time to time. Normal colds was the most common ailment, but it was stomach flu that really caused problems. Common symptoms are vomiting and diarrhea, and people who can smell usually find the smell of both activities extremely unpleasant, to say the least. My wife, who has a very sensitive sense of smell, gets sick herself from the smell. But in comes the anosmic husband as a superhero.

I especially remember one night when our son was about 4-5 years old. He felt really bad that evening so we put him to sleep in our bed at bedtime, with a bucket close at hand. He woke up in the middle of the night, I helped him to vomit in the bucket, comforted him, then put him back to sleep whereafter I could empty and clean the bucket. The procedure repeated itself about once every hour during most of the night, but around 5-6 in the morning everything finally calmed down and we could both relax and get some real sleep. My wife had moved to another room when everything started, knowing that she would not be of any help. That way she was rested when morning came and I could sleep a few extra hours.

So in times of sickness, the anosmic parent can be a real asset. But when the children bring home something with a nice scent they made in pre-school, you are lost. I can still remember the first time my son brought home something he had made. I took it, looked at it and said, "Nice, you're really clever" or something like that, like parents do. He looked at me, somewhat confused, and said, "You're supposed to smell it!" I explained to him that I could not smell anything. He looked surprised, and asked me if could not smell anything at all? When I said no, he

Being an anosmic parent

thought for a few seconds and simply said, "Okay" and that was it.

Both my children learned early on that I could not smell and to them it was just the way it was. There was nothing strange or weird about it. But even if they did not find my anosmia strange, even if they knew I was anosmic, they still forgot about it sometimes. My daughter would bake a cake or buy a scented soap and hold it for me to smell it, but remembering right then that I could not. But because my anosmia was so completely normal to both my children, those moments never became awkward.

Then they became teenagers.

I have heard anosmic parents express concern about the teenage years, with a particular worry about drugs. Being anosmic, there was no way I could tell if they smelled of alcohol or any other drug, but I was lucky. I had a wife who could, and due to her work she knew all about these things, and our children knew that she knew. So we were lucky and never had any serious problems.

And having children that could smell in a way gave me a new perspective on the concept–what are smells?

COMMENTS ABOUT SMELLS

FROM WHAT I have heard, the sense of smell is very special. It is very different compared to sight and taste, because it cannot be turned off. It is always active, but in a discreet way, in the background, often without people consciously noticing it. If I do not eat, I sense no taste, and if I close my eyes, the sight center of my brain can rest for a while. But the sense of smell never rests. In that way it resembles hearing, but sounds do not appear to affect people in the same way that smells do. People often comment on smells, and very often they do not seem to be consciously aware of it. It is usually neither questions nor answers, just general comments not directed at anyone in particular. And by doing this, they often unconsciously pass judgment on the room they enter, or a person they just passed.

For a person with anosmia these comments are conspicuous because they force me to think about smells. I never think about seeing or hearing, or tasting when I eat, but I am repeatedly forced to think about smells, in spite of not knowing what it is, because it is so important to everyone else.

Because the sense of smell is always active, always present, and cannot be turned off, even people who are really close to me, like parents, siblings, partner, and children, sometimes forget that I am anosmic. A common scenario is when someone smells something special and wants to share it:

"Oh, what a nice smell..." and then they hold the flower, or soap, or whatever it is that smells so nicely, under my nose. Or the opposite:

"Ouch, this xxx really smells bad" and then they stretch out their arm as far as possible and hold the item for me to smell. When I answer "Okay ...?" with a blank face they realize their mistake and often try to save the situation with a comment like:

"Well, you know, it smells like ..." and then they compare with ... another smell!

I think it is a bit funny that when people who can smell try to describe a smell to me, they often begin by referring to another smell. The next step is to compare with taste.

"It smells like, a combination of..." and then they may give an example of food or spices.

Although I could possibly imagine how such a combination would taste, I cannot transcribe it into anything else. The analogy that it smells like it tastes, but you feel it with your nose instead of your mouth, may be reasonable for someone who can smell, but not to me. I cannot imagine how I could feel the taste somewhere else than where the food is, in my mouth. The thought of stuffing food in my nose does not help me understand what smells are. On top of that, the taste they compare with is often unknown to me because what they perceive as taste is actually a flavor dominated by smells. So in the end they are again comparing with another smell.

I can think about what it would feel like to sense smells, from an intellectual, philosophical point of view but honestly, I have no clue. To me, sensing smells is as fictional as having x-ray sight, or being telepathic, or sensing the strength and direction of magnetic fields. Such things may exist in fairytales or in science-fiction novels, but not for real.

Another common comment is, "Surely you miss being able to smell?" To me that question is as strange as if I would counter by

Comments about smells

asking, "Surely you miss being able to read peoples minds?" or "Do you miss being able to sense magnetic fields?". No, I do not miss being able to sense something that does not exist, at least not in my world.

I do not walk around thinking about what smells could be present where I am, but which I cannot sense. Not even when I am writing this text about sensing smells am I thinking about smells because to me they do not exist. To me it is only words, something you write in texts, or talk about. When someone comments on how nice a flower smells, I hear the comment, but it does not really mean anything to me. It is only words.

This non-existence of smells in my world sometimes creates situations and moments that are quite absurd.

The absurd world of smells

A FEW DAYS before I wrote this I listened to the local radio station. They were discussing lavender. A woman explained how she made small bags of cloth, filled them with lavender, and then put them in her linen cupboards. I had to ask my wife what they were talking about. Why would you put lavender in cupboards. The people at the local radio station took for granted that everyone knew that lavender smells nice, and that it only takes a small amount to spread a nice smell in a cupboard. Getting this explanation I suddenly remembered having seen such bags in my parents house when I was a child, but I never understood the point of those small pouches.

A really absurd experience for an anosmic is when you enter a shop that sells perfume. The whole concept is incomprehensible to me. A whole store full of small bottles and jars filled with colored water that the customers open and hold under their noses, or dip small paper sticks in which they then wave around in front of their nose. To me the colored water in the bottles and jars is just that: colored water. Sometimes an employee helps my wife, and then politely offers to let me smell the samples as well. I often pretend to smell, not to be impolite. A fellow anosmic described how she, in a similar situation, politely told a saleswoman that she was anosmic and could not sense smells. This resulted in a scolding from the saleswoman who said that if the customer did not like the smell she only had to say so, instead of inventing some strange excuse.

Some of the bottles and jars apparently emit vapor that trigger the receptors of the trigeminal nerve. They often make the air in the shops feel irritating and unpleasant. To a person who can smell I suppose the nice smells override the irritating vapor, but to me they create an absurd experience. To me the perfume-shop becomes a place with really unpleasant air, where others walk around oblivious to this, smelling jars and bottles and saying "Aaahhh..." and "Mmm...".

And talking about perfume and such, deodorants are interesting in their own special way. Most of the anosmics I have been in touch with use deodorant on a daily basis, in spite of not knowing what they use. I do the same. So how do we know what to use? We simply do not, so we either just guess based on for example if it is a nice label, or we need advice from someone who can smell. But even if we have a nice smelling deodorant, we still do not know how much to use. A young female anosmic told a story about how she for several years had used a special deodorant which she thought smelled nice. Having had a new boyfriend for a while she one day asked him what he thought about it. He admitted that he really disliked it, but had been afraid to tell her. He had no idea that she was anosmic.

A good example of how congenital anosmics do not understand about smell, is the discussion we recently had in our Facebook group. One of the members asked if snow has a smell. There were strong opinions both pro and con, and some wild speculations about causes for yes or no. I asked my daughter, who gave a clear answer with a logical motivation: snow is pure water, pure water does not smell, so consequently snow does not smell. I took her answer and passed it on to the Facebook group where it triggered a reaction that is probably incomprehensible to anyone with a functioning sense of smell: "So water has no

The absurd world of smells

smell? Strange, I thought all liquids smelled". To me that response made total sense. We have learned that other liquids smell, that lakes and the sea smell, so why not pure water? For a congenital anosmic it is simply impossible to know what smells and what does not, and thus to know that pure water does not smell.

I once read a story which described our inability to understand smells in a beautiful way. It was about the congenitally anosmic wife who wanted to surprise her husband with a cake when he returned from work on his birthday. She made the cake in the afternoon and hid it to surprise him after dinner. Coming in through the front door, he immediately asked "Have you been baking?" The wife had no idea that smells could linger for several hours, so the element of surprise was gone. The following year she made the cake early in the morning, and kept doors and windows open all day, to get rid of the smell long before her husband came home. "Have you been baking?" was his first words when he opened the front door. The wife has continued to bake birthday cakes, but she gave up on trying to surprise him.

Both these stories are good examples of our inability to understand smells. There are obviously no simple rules for if and how different things smell, or for how long a smell will linger.

So how does my anosmia affect my day-to-day life?

PART TWO

LIFE WITH ANOSMIA

THE SENSE OF TASTE

THE MOST COMMON question I get when I tell someone that I have no sense of smell is probably "Can you taste?" To me that question is utterly incomprehensible. When I eat I sense the taste with my tongue, not with my nose, so why should smell have anything to do with taste? But for those that can smell it is a logical question. To understand why our experiences of taste are so different you need to understand how the sense of taste functions, and how tastes are created by the brain.

It is still a widely spread belief that there are only four basic tastes, sweet, salt, sour and bitter, and that different areas on the tongue sense each of these four basic tastes. Science has long since shown this to be wrong.

Almost the entire tongue is covered by papillae. Some of them contain the taste buds, the structures that register taste. Each taste bud consists of 50-100 taste cells, positioned roughly like the sections in an orange. These taste cells register the different tastes of what we eat. There are taste cells for all basic tastes in all taste buds, and therefore all taste buds can register all tastes.

Earlier it was believed that there were four basic tastes but some years ago 'umami' was added. It can be described as "meat taste". Researchers are also discussing if "fat" and "carbonation" should be classified as basic tastes, because receptors for these tastes have been identified. So in total there are five, six or seven basic tastes, or perhaps even more. With more research being done, I would not be surprised if the concept "basic tastes" will be redefined in the future.

In addition to the taste buds there are other receptors in the mouth, connected to the trigeminal nerve. Their function is to register the texture and shape of what we eat, but they can also register pain, heat, cold, and tingling. Some spices stimulate not only the taste buds but also, or even only, the trigeminal nerve cells.

Mint is registered by the trigeminal nerve as cold. If you taste a mint pastil and then inhale through your mouth, the brain will register that you inhaled air and that the receptors for cold were activated. So the brain connects the two and draws the conclusion that you inhaled cold air. That is the reason it feels cold when you inhale after eating cough drops, despite the fact that the air you are inhaling has exactly the same temperature as before you took the cough drop.

Mustard, pepper and onion can, in a similar way, activate receptors for heat and pain, which are also connected to the trigeminal nerve. That is why peppers can feel almost painfully strong and cause you to sweat. The brain is fooled to believe that it is warm.

Pain is a signal that is prioritized by the brain, so if there are simultaneous signals for pain and taste coming from the tongue, the brain more or less ignores the taste signals. Because of this, if I eat something with a lot of pepper in it, I sense almost no taste, only a burning sensation on the tongue and the mucous membranes in the mouth. This signal usually remains for a while, making it feel like the tongue is buzzing and the sense of taste is turned off.

I have a similar reaction with very warm food or drink. Hot food triggers the heat receptors of the trigeminal nerve, sending

The sense of taste

a strong signal to the brain warning for heat, resulting in a simultaneous blocking of the taste signals. As a result, I sense no taste from very hot coffee. It only burns and feels unpleasantly hot.

Some vegetables, like rhubarb, unripe fruit and some brands of tea, contain tannins which evoke a feeling or taste of harshness in the mouth. That taste is registered by the mucous membrane in the mouth and not the taste buds.

This describes the sense of taste in the way it works for me. It is a combination of taste registered by the taste buds and signals from the trigeminal nerve registering structure, heat, cold, pain and tingling. For people who can smell the smells sensed by the nose are added to this, so what they call taste is a combination of three different systems: the sense of taste, the sense of smell and the trigeminal nerve. Together it creates what could be called *flavor*. For a person with a functioning sense of smell, at least three quarters of the flavor they experience consist of smells. If such a person suddenly loses her ability to sense smells, she experiences that most of the flavor disappears. Some say that it disappears completely, some that it is reduced to the five basic tastes sweet, salt, sour, bitter and umami. To prove that this is true for a person who can smell, all you have to do is to pinch your nose, hold your breath and taste something, or compare how food tastes if you have a severe cold with a stuffed nose.

Does this mean that I, being born anosmic, cannot experience a multitude of tastes? No, that is wrong. I have a well developed sense of taste and can recognize even small differences in taste, and many of the congenital anosmics I have been in touch with claim the same. How is that possible?

ANOSMIC TASTE

SMELL IS A very complicated phenomenon, and the brain consequently dedicates a rather large part of its capacity to handling input from the olfactory system. But if you are a congenital anosmic the brain never gets any such input. This might influence the way the brain develops when you are a child. Without olfactory input the whole "smell center" in the brain is free for other tasks. Knowing that smell and taste input are processed in the same area of the brain, it is possible that the brain of a congenital anosmic uses a larger part of the brain for analyzing taste input than the brain does for a person who can smell. If so, for a congenital anosmic the taste input from the tongue would be processed and analyzed in a more advanced way. This could explain why congenital anosmics often perceive a more refined taste than acquired anosmics do. But there is more to it.

Taste is by definition restricted to what we sense with taste buds, but because the tongue is also covered by receptors of the trigeminal nerve, I cannot separate what I sense with my taste buds from what I sense with my trigeminal nerve. Everything is connected. And because trigeminal nerve cells also register texture, I usually experience texture as part of the taste. Consequently, a piece of apple does not taste apple in the same way as apple juice.

Furthermore, when I taste something, all signals coming from the different taste and trigeminal receptors are usually blended, creating one taste. In a way it is like colors. Just like mixing various colors creates one shade of color, mixing different ingredients and spices creates one shade of taste.

This also explains why congenital anosmics seldom can identify exactly what ingredients were included to create a specific taste, in the same way that it afterwards is impossible to say exactly which colors an artist mixed to create one resulting shade. But there is one exception. Because taste and texture are connected, I can usually separate the taste of ingredients that have very different texture, even when mixed in the same bite. The tastes of potatoes, steak and gravy can usually be separated even if I mix them in the same bite.

Continuing the analogy with vision, humans can distinguish numerous shades of color, but we do not have common names for every single shade. We only have names for a few basic colors. If we are presented with two slightly different shades, we can clearly see that there is a difference. If we are only presented with one of them, we cannot decide for sure which one it is, but we can definitely say which basic color it leans towards.

It is the same thing with sound. Humans can distinguish lots of different tones and timbres, but very few can identify single notes. In spite of this most people can appreciate music.

My sense of taste works in analogy to this. I can sense the difference between slightly different shades of taste if presented with both, I can say which basic taste they lean towards, but I can seldom identify the ingredients used to blend that shade of taste. Even so, I can still appreciate the taste of what I am eating.

A common objection is that it is impossible to have a refined sense of taste because there are only a few basic tastes. That is true but again we can use the analogy of colors. A laser printer can create millions of color shades with four color toners and a

Anosmic taste

white paper. Surely it should be possible to create, if not millions at least a few thousand, different shades of taste by combining the five, six or seven basic tastes and the input from the trigeminal nerve? That an acquired anosmic, with an untrained sense of taste, cannot do it does not prove that it cannot be done. I know it can be done, because I experience it daily, every time I eat.

A problem in this context is that most scientific taste studies are done on persons with acquired anosmia and smell is used as the norm to which taste is compared. Almost everyone with a functioning sense of smell can identify thousands of individual smells and they all have names. Honey, rose, tulip, buttercup, wet dog, wet earth, sea weed, lavender, rosemary, sage, thyme, wool, and so on. When congenital anosmics are tested, a common mistake is to perform the tests as identification tests, testing if anosmics can identify different food stuff as well as someone with a functioning sense of smell. As I explained above, we cannot do that. The sense of taste does not work like that, but this does not mean we cannot distinguish between two tastes when presented with both.

If we return to the analogy with the laser printer, many of us with congenital anosmia possibly have a sense of taste with a very high resolution, while people who were born with a functioning sense of smell have a sense of taste with low resolution. But then again, there is also considerable variation within the group of congenital anosmics. I asked the members of our Facebook group how they would rate their sense of taste. About half of them claimed to have a well developed sense of taste, being able to separate between very similar tastes. The other half described their sense of taste as limited. Some even described their experience as having almost no sense of taste, which resembles how acquired anosmics describe their sense of taste.

Lars Lundqvist

One way to describe the difference in sense of taste between acquired and congenital anosmics is to compare it with other senses. I once read the following analogy, suggested by a fellow congenital anosmic. Flavor could be compared with a movie, where the picture represented smell and the sound taste. A person with both eyesight and hearing would focus on the visual part of the movie, the visible story, while much of the music and other sounds would be registered subconsciously. If this person suddenly lost her eyesight, the person would hear the same sounds, but most of all be acutely aware of not seeing the pictures. A congenitally blind person would be used to focusing all her attention on hearing the sounds, and would probably hear details which the person with acquired blindness would miss.

So, being a congenital anosmic I have a brain where the whole smell center is free, making it possible for five, six, seven or even more basic tastes, to combine with receptors for texture, cold, heat, pain and harshness. It should not come as a surprise that I can feel a large spectrum of tastes, in spite of not having a sense of smell.

So what are the differences between the tastes someone who can smell and I experience?

Food and anosmia

FOR SOME FOODS there is probably almost no difference between the taste you experience with or without a sense of smell. For other things there is a tremendous difference. Things like sugar lumps, ordinary salt, perhaps lemon juice and other food stuff with only one very distinct basic taste and very little smell, probably taste roughly the same to me and a person who can smell. But the more smell something contains, the larger the difference in what we experience. To me garlic is perhaps the most extreme example.

Fresh garlic creates a rather sharp sensation for me, without any clear taste, unlike for example white pepper, which also creates the sharp sensation, but which also has a very specific taste. Furthermore, garlic is not very strong compared to black or white pepper, so I need quite a lot of raw garlic to taste the presence of garlic in a sauce or tzatziki. One clove does not do much good. If garlic is heated in a dish, like a warm sauce or roast lamb, even the sharp sensation disappears. To me the garlic disappears completely, without leaving any trace. But if you instead marinate garlic in olive oil, most of the sharp sensation disappears, and the taste of the garlic suddenly appears and is amplified, making it taste deliciously. It then tastes so good that I happily eat clove after clove, but this usually provokes complaints from my family. They claim that my breath smells of garlic afterwards, and apparently it is not a nice smell.

Herbs used as spices in food are another example where the experiences of anosmics and those that can smell are completely different. Most herbs affect the flavor of a dish through smell and not through taste. Hence, I seldom notice the herbs in food. For some herbs it is possible to elicit the taste by marinating the herb in oil, but even then it usually requires a fairly large amount of the herb, like when you make pesto.

Nowadays it is common for foods to have some extra taste added, like olive oil with a hint of lemon or tea spiced with herbs. However, for most of these flavored foods it is not a taste that has been added, but a smell. If you read the description carefully it usually says that an aromatic has been added, and those aromatics are usually volatile substances that only emit smells, not taste. The flavored food is thus smell enhanced, not taste enhanced. As a result, to an anosmic like me the flavored food tastes just like an unflavored version. I cannot sense the flavoring.

Candy is a typical example of smell enhanced flavored foodstuff. Pears taste like pears, and apples like apples, but pear and apple jelly usually only taste like sweet jelly without any hint of pear or apple. There is usually no difference in taste between differently colored candies although they may be made to mimic different fruits. The explanation is again that the flavors are volatile aromatics, basically only changing the smell and not the taste of the candy.

Another difference in how we perceive taste is related to how the sense of smell reacts to constant stimuli. If a person who can smell enters a room with a strong odor, she will not sense the odor after a while. The sense of smell gradually adapts itself to the odor, a phenomenon called olfactory fatigue or olfactory adaption. This phenomenon also manifests itself when you are eating, and it has been studied by scientists. If someone who can smell eats bite after bite of something very delicious, she will appreciate the bites slightly less for each bite she eats, and after many bites, the final bite will not be nearly as tasty as the first. The sense of smell gets tired rather quickly, and diminishes the flavor over time.

The sense of taste also gradually adapts itself, but at a much slower rate than the sense of smell. In the studies done, the scientists found that congenital anosmics thought that the first and last bite tasted almost the same, and almost equally good. I can corroborate this being exactly the way it is for me. The other day my family and I were eating straw berries, and there were plenty to eat. The others ate some strawberries each and then they did not want anymore. The tenth strawberry did not taste as good as the first one. But I kept eating, until we ran out of strawberries, and just like the results in the study I thought that the first and the last strawberry were almost equally tasty.

As I mentioned before, pain and heat signals from the trigeminal nerve are prioritized by the brain. The sense of smell can usually register any spices present as flavors but, obviously, I cannot. Instead my sense of taste is being almost totally blocked out by the overwhelming signals from the trigeminal nerve. Therefore, I usually avoid food that is very spicy or very hot. Tepid and mildly spiced food usually tastes best for me.

So how does all this affect my food preferences and how I eat? The basic principle can be summarized as "not too warm and, one thing at a time and big wet bites".

Hot coffee apparently smells very nice, but for me to taste it, it needs to cool a bit. Adding a little milk reduces the temperature and neutralizes some of the bitterness. Adding a sugar lump or two makes it taste even nicer, so I want my coffee white and sweet.

'Not too warm' applies also to food. When everyone else starts eating instantly, the second the food is on the plate, I have to wait for the temperature to drop a bit. Sometimes the result is that everyone else has more or less finished their meal before I have even begun eating.

Mixing textures and tastes feels weird and sometimes distorts the taste for me so I usually prefer to eat one thing at a time. At the restaurant at my work they have a salad bar with a lot of different mixed salads. My colleagues appear to really like it and praise its quality. To me it is almost the ultimate horror. Although the salads often contain ingredients I really like, it is impossible to separate them, so to me the result is an impossible mix of textures and tastes, creating a chaos of taste signals so nothing tastes the way it is supposed to do. On top of that the salads often contain ingredients that have almost no taste at all, only texture, like most kinds of beans, rice, cold pasta, couscous, bulgur, etcetera. The only solution for me is to pick specific things in the salads, like big pieces of tomato, cauliflower, broccoli or artichoke, or some coleslaw. For some reason coleslaw is okay. I guess it is because of the very distinct taste of vinegar, which I really like.

I really dislike sweet food with a gooey texture. Two typical examples are cheesecake and chocolate pudding. I have received similar opinions from other anosmics, and have actually seen it confirmed in a scientific study performed some decades ago. My guess is that there are two explanations for this. First, the texture feels unpleasant, and secondly and perhaps more important, it feels as if the sweet gooey texture causes an overload on the taste buds. For someone who can smell the smell component probably is so strong that it dominates completely, and maybe the high load on the badly trained taste buds just add an extra taste sensation?

There is another big difference between smell and taste. It only takes a small amount of a substance to produce a scent and

Food and anosmia

thus create a flavor that a person with a sense of smell can perceive. My sense of taste does not work that way at all. To properly taste something, I need a big bite to activate a sufficient number of taste buds to get a really good reading of how it tastes. There are taste buds not only on the tongue but also in the soft part of the palate, so I taste with my whole mouth. And if it is something I find delicious, the bigger the bite, the more delicious it tastes. Furthermore, the food has to be moist or wet to activate the taste buds properly. Dry food usually has very little or no taste. Because of this I usually take a sip of whatever I am drinking together with every bite, before I start chewing.

Finally, because smell is such a large part of the flavor experienced by a person who can smell, the flavor can be affected by smells originating in the surroundings, not connected to the food. So even the most delicious meal might taste weird or even really bad if eaten in a stinking environment. This, obviously, is not the case for me. To me a specific dish will always taste the same, irrespective of where I eat it. In the kitchen, on a beach, or on a garbage dump. And when I eat the Swedish specialty "surströmming," fermented herring, it is an advantage not to be bothered by the smell.

But not being able to smell my surroundings or the food I eat may actually cause danger in my day-to-day life.

Bad food

I GUESS THAT you have seen a parent, sibling, friend or partner take something from the refrigerator, sniff it and then exclaim "Yuk, this is inedible". No one has ever seen me do that. I look at the date on the milk pack and when the Best before-date has passed I avoid even tasting it. I have occasionally forgotten to check the date and, unprepared, gotten a mouthful of sour milk. It is not something I would recommend. It tastes horribly.

It is the same thing with bread. My wife sniffs the bread and says, "It smells of mold" which means I do not eat it. If she is not around, there are only three alternatives. To trust the date on the package, to scrutinize every slice of bread for signs of mold, or risk suddenly discovering mold on the piece of half-eaten bread still left in my hand. When we buy bread from a bakery or bake it ourselves there is no date, so then the only alternative is to try to remember the age of the bread and to scrutinize for mold. If I am unsure, I refrain from eating it and throw it away. At the same time throwing food away feels a bit stupid because to me there is nothing wrong with the bread, ham, sausage, etcetera. They appear to be all right and usually also taste okay, but I know that I might still get sick from eating it.

I am not alone feeling this concern of whether the food is edible or perhaps unhealthy to eat. I have heard the same story from many anosmics, and even stories of anosmics hit by food poisoning due to not knowing that the food had been saved for too long. A person who can smell would have noticed the strange smell coming from the food and thrown it away. Being anosmic I have to rely on sight and taste, and food can be quite unhealthy before tasting bad or even slightly different from its ordinary taste.

In some restaurants you are expected to test the wine before it is served. I never understood the point of doing this (am I allowed to choose another wine if I do not like it, or what am I expected to test?) so I usually try to let someone else test it. But then, on one occasion, I finally understood the point of testing it. My wife lifted her glass to her mouth but hesitated, sniffed the wine a little, then asked to sniff the cork and the bottle, before stating that, "It does not smell the way it should," and the wine was replaced.

This ability that others have, to be able to say, "It does not smell as it should" can sometimes appear almost magical, because it is so utterly incomprehensible to me. My wife takes something from the refrigerator, meaning to use it for dinner, but suddenly stops and says "It doesn't smell the way it should" and throws it away. When I look at it, I cannot see anything separating it from other similar foodstuff that smells okay. To me there is absolutely no difference whatsoever! If I had been alone, I would probably have eaten it without noticing anything peculiar about it and possibly have turned ill.

The only solution for me is to have complete faith in the Best-before dates. But there is a problem. For some foodstuff the date is only valid provided you do not open the packaging. If you are lucky, it says something on the label about how long the food remains edible after opening the package, which at least gives you a chance to memorize when you opened it or to write a date on the packaging. But usually there is nothing like that. You are expected to be able to smell the condition of the opened package

Bad food

which means I haven't got a chance.

So how do I handle it? I do just as I do with so many other things; I follow simple rules.

LIVING BY RULES

NOT BEING ABLE to smell means I am not bothered by how things smell, or by how other humans smell. But ever since I was a child I have had to learn that to people who can smell, smells are really important and there are a lot of social conventions on how to handle smells. Somewhat simplified you could say that nobody and nothing is expected to smell dirty. Not you, not your cloths, not your home, not your office. To accomplish this, people frequently wash and clean everything. But clean is not enough. It has to smell nice too. So they use scented soap, shampoo and detergents.

Humans are trained to follow the smell conventions since childhood, so following the rules is second nature for a normal adult. A person who does not follow the smell conventions is seen as different, a bit strange, asocial or outright unpleasant.

To me smells do not exist but this does not mean that I can forget about smell conventions. Because smells are so important to everyone else I have to adapt myself and my behavior so that I do not provoke people around me and break their rules. My only option is to memorize things that smell, and when, and how much, and in what situations it matters. A strange consequence of my anosmia is thus that I have to think consciously about smells several times every day. Are my clothes smelling of sweat? Have I eaten something that gives me bad breath? How does my hair smell? This creates a constant stress.

Lars Lundqvist

The only way to handle this is to have rules. Simple, clear rules that are easy to remember and follow. Rules about clothes. Rules about cleaning. Rules about washing. Rules about personal hygiene. Rules about handling garbage. Rules and rules and rules. As long as I follow all these rules I should be on the safe side, not breaking any smell conventions, not provoking anyone, not behaving like a misfit.

Brushing my teeth after breakfast and before bedtime. Taking a shower, using deodorant and putting on clean underwear and shirt before going to work. Taking a shower if I have been sweating. Those things you do every day or which are easily connected to a specific activity are fairly easy to understand and remember, but after that it becomes more complicated.

Clothes and smell are a difficult combination. To me it does not matter if a t-shirt is freshly washed or if I have been wearing it every day during the last week. It feels the same to me. But it matters to people who can smell. Intellectually I can understand that when I work so hard that my t-shirt gets all sweaty, it will smell. Although the t-shirt feels the same once it is dry again, I can rationally understand how someone with a sense of smell would perceive the t-shirt. But what about socks? Do I have to change socks every day, or does it depend on what I have done during the day, if I have been wearing shoes all day or not, and if so what kind of shoes? And trousers are even more difficult. How often do I have to wash my jeans or chinos? I seldom sweat so profoundly that they get wet from sweat, so how can they become so dirty that they smell just by me wearing them?

Of course I have learned that clothes slowly get dirty when you use them, even if they do not become visibly stained. So intellectually and theoretically I understand the concept and process. But emotionally, deep down, I do not understand at all, because I have never experienced how dirt smells. Therefore, it is essentially impossible for me to decide when it is time to wash trousers. There is no simple rule to follow, so I just have to guess, or ask my wife.

I am lucky enough to have a wife who can help me with everyday chores, but it is still a problem because I do not always understand the answers I get. If I ask her "Does this shirt smell" and I get the answer "Yes, a little" I have no idea how to interpret it. It does not tell me anything about how others see me if I use that shirt. Not knowing what smell is, I know even less about differences in levels of smells. And this is made even more complicated by the fact that the sensitivity of the sense of smell differs among people: each person has a different opinion about nice and bad smells.

I recently discussed this problem with clothes and smell with close relatives. I explained the problem of not knowing when certain types of clothes should be washed, like trousers and sweaters. They tried to reassure me that it is no problem, because such items seldom need to be washed, and in between they can be aired from time to time to make them feel a bit fresher. To me this is a perfect example of how they do not understand that I do not understand. Their explanation does not make it any easier. Is "seldom" once a month or once a year? How many days can you wear trousers before you have to wash them? Five days, ten days, fifty days, a hundred days? Without someone to smell things for me, the only way to avoid clothes smelling is to wash everything at frequent intervals, whether someone who can smell would think it was necessary or not. Better safe than sorry.

And then there are all those things that are hard to regulate, like changing towels and bed linen, vacuuming the house, scrubbing the floors, and so on.

A congenital anosmic who has cats told me how she worries all the time that her cats or their litter box will smell badly. What will visitors think? Is the smell a problem, or is there no reason to worry? Because she cannot tell if the cats or the litter box smell at all, her only option is to rely on others to help her.

Another good example of how my smell-free world sometimes collides with the world of people who can smell, is house cleaning. My wife and I try to share the responsibilities for household work as fairly as possible, but house cleaning has always been a problem. Why? Because something being dirty is more a question of smells than of looks.

Intellectually I understand the principles about dirt and cleanliness, that you have to vacuum the house, scrub the floors and dust bookshelves and other furniture, but I have no emotional connection to it. Entering a room I might notice that there is litter on the floor, or that hair balls from our dog or cats are whirling in a corner, but the room basically feels clean. When my wife enters the same room, she might say that it feels stale, dirty, not fresh, and it is basically a question of how it smells. And this is where the problems start.

My world is essentially always clean. A room may be disorganized, littered, but never dirty in the sense it is perceived if you can smell. And because I never really experience any room as dirty there is never really any reason to clean it. It is already clean! So again I have to have a set of rules to handle this. But how do you keep rules for things that happen very seldom? How often do you need to scrub the floors? Or wipe dust? The longer the interval, the harder it is to have a rule. How often do you need to wash a tablecloth? Only if it has stains, or also when it has been used quite a while but has no stains? And what about curtains? Should you wash curtains, and if so how often, or seldom? Or carpets? Do you need to wash carpets?

Unfortunately it seems that the only reliable answer to all those questions is "It depends...". On what? On whether they are dirty or not, and the only way to decide if they are dirty enough to need cleaning is by smelling them. Which means that I have lost the game before it even started.

Rules—a blessing and a curse

FOLLOWING RULES IS not unique for me as an anosmic. Everyone else of course also have to follow the same set of rules. But there is a big difference. I have no idea to what degree the rules make me succeed or not in following the smell conventions. With a sense of smell you can take a sniff and say, "I wore this t-shirt yesterday but it smells okay so I can wear it again today". I cannot do that. I have to follow the rules, blindly, or risk making a serious mistake. And although I have memorized a lot of rules, being anosmic I really do not know the difference between following or not following a specific rule. What is the difference in smell between a newly washed t-shirt and one that I wore several days? I have no idea.

And although the rules are meant to make my life easier and help me to follow social conventions, they simultaneously add a constant stress to my life. I usually do not think about the rules, because I usually do not think about smells, so I consciously have to remind myself, over and over, not to forget them. Consciously or unconsciously I am constantly waiting for comments about smells. Comments that will tell me if I have succeeded in following all the social smell-rules or not.

Sometimes comments about smells are expressed as questions, making everything even more irritating and stressful.

"What is that smell, is it...?" followed by an example of something that apparently smells.

Lars Lundqvist

Although I can intellectually understand that it is a rhetorical question, such questions always feel unfair. Subconsciously they are felt like criticism, accusing me of being too dumb to understand smells. But how could I? It is like criticizing a congenitally blind person for not having changed a broken light bulb. How could a congenitally blind person even understand what a light bulb is? A person who has never experienced light cannot understand the difference between light and dark, and it is the same for me regarding smells. I have no conception of what it is.

All this is creating a constant low level stress. And even if I do my best to remember the rules, my lack of understanding sometimes make me fail to follow the smell conventions.

One feeling when I fail is resignation. Why bother? It feels pointless to even try because I have no way of knowing when I succeed or fail. It is so utterly unfair. Because no matter how hard I try, sooner or later I *will* fail, because I do not know what I am doing. I am only guessing.

The thing is, I never really think about smells. I have learned that I need to remember to think about it in certain situations, like when I have done something that made me sweat. But even then I really only think about the rules, not about smells.

The rules are meant as a tool to help me behave as if I had a sense of smell, to handle the smells that are so important to people around me but non-existing in my anosmic world. When the rules work, they not only help me to behave like someone who can smell but also emphasize the fact that I am different, a freak. I really try to follow them, but it is stressing to constantly have to remember all the rules, and every time I forget a rule I am reminded of being different. So ignoring the rules, not taking a shower, not changing possibly stinking clothes, is in a way a silent protest, a way of not accepting my being different. Disregarding

Rules—a blessing and a curse

the rules actually make me feel more normal, in my own smell-free world.

So living by rules is simultaneously both good and bad, a blessing and a curse, a help and an insult. So it should come as no surprise that on top of creating stress, my anosmia can also result in a stored anger and frustration.

ANGER

ALTHOUGH I AM anosmic, I am constantly pretending that I actually can smell and that I understand the concept. I do this so that I can take part in the social game at work, with neighbors, and so on. Would it not be easier just to tell everyone that I cannot sense smells? No, it would only create more stress, forcing me to answer the same questions, over and over again, explaining why I cannot smell and the consequences in everyday life.

Every time I tell someone that I am anosmic a whole cluster of questions are fired towards me:

"Can't you feel anything?" (no...)

"Not even very strong smells?" (no, a blind person can't see things just because they are big, right..?)

"But how can you taste?" (I have a tongue)

"Don't you miss being able to smell?" (how can I miss something which I don't know what it is?)

"When did you lose your sense of smell?" (I didn't...)

"Have you never been able to smell?" (no...)

"Have you always been like this?" (yes...)

"It does not show..." (no, how could it?)

"Why haven't you said this earlier?" (... so I wouldn't have to answer all these questions!)

On top of that, people always forget that I am anosmic, although I have told them, resulting in awkward situations when I remind them.

"What's that smell?" (I don't know...)

"Don't you smell it?" (no, I am anosmic, can't smell, remember? I told you yesterday...)

"Yeah, but surely you can smell this, when it's such a strong smell??"

... and all the questions start again. Or else you get an apologizing "Oh, sorry, I forgot..." and when you have experienced that a number of times, you stop reminding people. It is simply easier to say, "Yeah..." or "Mmm..." or "No idea..." and just ignore it. My life gets easier to live if I avoid the issue and just play along in the game, pretending that I can smell. At the same time this means that I am constantly hiding who I really am.

Another part of the anger and stress has to do with having to ask for help, being forced to ask others to smell yesterdays' shirt, food, and so on. I do not know if I am asking someone to smell something that is pleasant or unpleasant and presenting someone with something that really stinks is seldom appreciated. And having to ask for help with something that does not even exist in my world feels rather humiliating after a while.

And deep down there is probably some kind of anger about being anosmic. Why do people constantly demand that I think about something I do not understand? Why do they constantly have to remind me that I do not understand what smell is? Why should I constantly have to care about how others are affected by smells? Why should I constantly have to ask for help to handle all this?

So beyond being a very hands-on, daily problem, anosmia can also cause stress, frustration and anger. And sometimes a great sadness.

Sorrow

BOTH MY WIFE, my children, my siblings and my parents can smell. In fact, as far as I know, everyone around me can: colleagues, neighbors, relatives, friends. The big sadness in my life is that I can never share that dimension of their lives. I can never give my wife a compliment on how nice she smells and never give her perfume as a present. I could of course ask someone else to select a good perfume, but I would not really be able to share her joy over the present, because I honestly would not know what I was giving her. It might just as well be colored water. It would be as if a congenitally blind person would give someone a painting as a present.

There is no point in denying that there is a sadness in this: not really understanding what others talk about and constantly being reminded about not understanding. On top of that there is also a constant inner conflict. Should I inform everyone about my anosmia every time someone mentions smells, and again have to answer a lot of questions, or should I continue the game I learned as a kid, to play along and pretend? This second alternative is of course easier, but it means that I am hiding who I really am, and pretend to be something that I am not.

At the same time I do not wish I was someone or something else. Although there is a sadness deep inside, my anosmia is a part of me. This is the way I am, and I like my life and who I am. I do not know of any other way that life could potentially be because this is the only life I have lived and experienced. A life and a world where smells do not exist, except as words. So there is an inner conflict, between the desire to be accepted the way I am, and a wish to share the world that the people around me experience.

Of course there are times I wish I could, somehow, at least for a few minutes, share the reality my family experiences, and not be excluded from it.

Because I really am excluded! Although I cannot experience smells myself, I can get an indirect experience from your stories. That way I can understand that you have the privilege of experiencing something that I never will. Nowadays there are a lot of shows on TV about food, cooking, chefs, baking, etcetera, and in all those shows they use spices, they sniff food, and all participants talk about the different shades of wonderful smells and flavors that are blended. Seeing and listening to this, it becomes clear to me that there is a large dimension of life that I cannot experience.

But the sadness is not really about not being able to smell, about the sense of smell itself. It is about not being able to understand this thing you talk about, no matter how much I would want to. And it feels unfair, very sad, and very lonely. Because in the same way that I cannot share or understand your smelling world, you cannot share or understand my smell-free world. You can never understand, deep down, what it is like to live in a world without smells, and you cannot even understand that I do not understand your world.

And this is probably what hurts the most, what saddens me the most. This despair of never really being understood by people around me. That they never really understand that I do not know what smells are. No matter how hard I try to memorize all the rules, and try to behave correctly, I simply do not know what they are talking about. For them this thing 'smell' is so natural and so obvious, and that is why they cannot understand how utterly incomprehensible it is to me, with my congenital anosmia.

So sometimes I would just like to shout: I do not understand what you are talking about! I am just pretending! And I have been pretending all my life!

But being anosmic is not only a sorrow at times, it can also be quite dangerous.

FIRE AND OTHER DANGERS

FIRE IS A special subject for many anosmics. Not being able to sense the smell of smoke makes fire a serious concern. The only solution is to have smoke detectors. This is not unique for anosmics, but many anosmics have installed more smoke detectors than other people do, just to feel safe. Particularly when they live alone. Smoke detectors are our only way of getting an early warning of something happening that might turn into a fire.

I have a wife with a very well developed sense of smell, and she usually functions as a preliminary smoke detector. But I have realized that I have a complete trust in the smoke detectors' ability to detect smoke. When my wife suddenly says that she can smell smoke, I usually check if the smoke detectors are working. If everything looks all right, I simply assume that it is coming from elsewhere, like from a neighbor grilling meat.

But it is nevertheless a problem, because if someone in the family says that it smells of smoke, something must actually be burning or smoldering somewhere in the vicinity. The question is: where? Outside or indoors? I am of no help in locating the origin of the smell, and it could actually be dangerous even if it is coming from outside.

One spring day a few years ago my wife sensed the smell of smoke. It was not coming from inside, so she went out to identify the source. It was a neighbor burning old grass and twigs. It would not have been a problem, except the old man had not noticed that the fire had begun to spread behind him. With help from other neighbors the fire was extinguished before it had reached the closest buildings. But had I been home alone that day, I would probably not have noticed anything until the neighbor's old barn had been on fire.

Problems may also arise in spite of, or because of, having smoke detectors. Some time ago a smoke detector started screaming in the middle of the day. I was upstairs but rushed down, scared there was a fire. It was the detector inside the entrance that screamed. I saw no smoke and saw nothing that could have activated the detector, so I took it down and removed the battery to silence it. I looked it over and then put the battery back, which made it go off again. So I fetched the smoke detector from the living room to check the hallway, and nothing happened. It stayed quiet. The first one turned out to be malfunctioning. Luckily my wife was home that day, and she could tell me early on that it did not smell of smoke anywhere. Otherwise it would have been really scary because how would I else have known which smoke detector was functioning properly? The one that was silent or the one warning of a fire?

There is a type of modern smoke detectors which communicate with each other so that if one senses smoke, all of them sound the alarm. The logic behind this is that you should get the warning irrespective of where you are in a building, even if you are far from the fire. And being warned you can always locate the origin of the alarm by locating the room where it smells of smoke. Except that I cannot do that. To me this kind of communicating smoke detectors could create disaster, because I have no way of identifying the source of the alarm unless I see fire or smoke. Public buildings, like the university where I work, always have these communicating detectors so if there is smoke in one end, the alarm goes off everywhere. This makes it rather

Fire and other dangers

scary for me.

The most awkward situation is probably when someone, who does not know that I am anosmic, suddenly smells smoke and asks me if I also smell it. What am I supposed to answer? I cannot say "No," because in that situation there is usually no time for an explanation that I am anosmic and how my anosmia prevents me from smelling anything. When I was younger I often tried to evade the question by answering "Yes, maybe..?" but nowadays I usually give the truthful answer "I don't know" or "I've no idea". It usually results in a surprised face, and often the question is repeated and I give the same answer.

Another detail about my relation to fire, that is perhaps connected to my anosmia, is that I never light candles. Why? Mostly because I do not want to risk forgetting them, but also because I do not really see the point with candles. You get an extra point of light, but that is all. I have been told that there are scented candles, and that burning candles apparently can eliminate odors, but neither of these have any meaning to me.

Although fire is the big area of concern, there are other instances when my anosmia may cause concern. One such area is my car. If a passenger mentions a burning smell, I cannot identify it. Is it from the car or from outside, and if from the car then what is the source of the smell? Maybe something is overheating, but how would I know what it is, and how could I locate it? If I were alone in the car, I would not notice it at all until the car broke down.

It would be the same in the case of a fuel leak. I would not be aware of it unless it was streaming out from the car, being visible on the ground. However, fluids streaming from the car are not necessarily fuel. In the summer I often see a fluid streaming out from under the parked car. Nowadays I assume that it is water from the air-conditioning, but the first time it happened I did not know what it was. Water from the radiator? Gasoline? The only way for me to find out what it was would have been to taste it, but who wants to taste gasoline? So all I could do to try identify the liquid's origin was to touch it and see if it had a color.

Gas is a constant risk for anosmics as gas is unhealthy to inhale and leaking gas is explosive. A foul smelling component (mercaptan, which apparently smells like rotten egg) is sometimes added to the gas, to warn for leaks. But that does not help anosmics. Gas detectors are available, just like smoke detectors, but I have heard of several anosmics who for this reason use electric appliances instead.

Fire, unknown liquids and gas are only a few examples of things that are difficult to handle for an anosmic. To handle these and other dangers and difficulties we need help.

Help me!

HOW DO PEOPLE react if I tell them that I am anosmic? Do they ask me if I need any help and if so how they can help? No, that is extremely unusual. Instead there are some standard reactions that probably almost all anosmics have encountered.

The most common reactions are probably the questions that express surprise, such as "Can you taste?" "How long have you been like this?" However, when the questions have been answered the conversation continues as before and is soon about something completely different. And then, after a while, the person suddenly will ask you to smell something. Either that person did not listen to your answers, or did not understand, or simply forgot. In either case it is rather frustrating to me.

Then we have those who answer with what they think is a funny comment, like "Lucky you! Then you won't have to smell..." followed by a joke about someone or something that smells really bad. I find this behavior insulting. It is similar to saying to a blind person "Lucky you're blind, because xxx is really ugly". The only logical explanation for this kind of reaction is that the person does not understand how important the sense of smell really is, even to himself.

Sometimes the listener reacts with distrust and suspicion. "Can't you sense any smells at all? Not even very strong ones?" The issue is then dismissed as something both weird and unimportant. This reaction is, surprisingly, rather common from medical doctors throughout the world. The only time I mentioned my anosmia to a doctor his response was "Well, bad for you..." and then shifted the conversation to something completely different.

Finally we have those who react with seriousness and thoughtfulness. "Wow, that's really interesting..." followed by reflections and comments about how difficult it is to understand what it means. This is the reaction I prefer. It is encouraging in the sense that it shows that the other person is listening, trying to understand. An inevitable consequence obviously is that it simultaneously amplifies the feeling that I really do not understand smells or what it is that I am missing.

So what should you do if you can smell and have a congenital anosmic among people close to you, such as a child, a sibling, a parent, a partner, a friend, a colleague. What can you do to facilitate the life of the anosmic? There are three simple things:

<u>The first</u> and most important is that you remember that the person is anosmic.

Being born without a sense of smell I constantly have to learn, memorize and follow rules and routines connected to smells: take a shower when I have worked up a sweat, use deodorant, think about my breath, remember to take out the garbage, make sure I have clean non-smelling clothes, and so on. I do this to not offend your sensitive noses, and so does every anosmic. In return we would appreciate if at least you would remember that we are anosmic so we will not have to repeat ourselves.

That people around me have such a hard time remembering my anosmia is probably partly a result of congenital anosmia being rather unusual and unnoticed in our society, and partly because people in general are unaware of how often they refer to smells. But being anosmic it is very frustrating that so many around me, even family members, have such a hard time remembering that I am anosmic.

The second is to lend us your nose when we ask for it.

If I ask if a shirt smells of sweat it is not because I am curious about the smell itself. It is only because I want to know if I can use it one more day. And you have to make that decision for me, because I cannot. I have nothing to compare it with and consequently cannot even have an opinion. So you must have the courage to make my decision.

It is the same if I ask if the milk, or the ham, or some other foodstuff smells okay so I can eat it. It is not to get a second opinion. I just want you to do the smell test that I cannot do. And again, you have to make the decision.

Another anosmic described a situation where she was in desperate need of a nose. She discovered that a pillow in the sofa was wet at one end, and also the cushion under it. But what kind of fluid was it? Had someone just spilled some water, or had the dog urinated on it? If it was water, it was not a problem. She could wait until the sofa was dry again. But if it was dog pee, the pillow and cushion had to be cleaned. Without a sense of smell it was impossible to decide what kind of fluid it was, except if you tasted it. But who would want to check it if it might be dog pee?

The third is to be tolerant and accept our failures. When we make a wrong decision, or forget one of the many smell-rules, it is not because we do not care, but because we do not notice the difference. Accept our failures and avoid pointing it out in a criticizing way.

I know that smells are important for people who can smell, so if you feel you have to tell me about what you smell, it is okay. However, it is useless to phrase it as a question because that implies I can answer, and I cannot. If I or my clothes are smelling of sweat, and you think I should take a shower or change clothes, tell me politely. Do not hint that I should know this myself because I really cannot.

As a fellow anosmic phrased it: Telling an anosmic that she stinks is like telling a blind person that her clothes are ugly.

So, three points:

1) Remember that a person is anosmic.

2) Lend us your nose when we ask for it.

3) Accept our failures.

Apart from these three there is one more general understanding to remember, especially if you are a parent with an anosmic child.

Smells do not exist to a person with congenital anosmia.

I have stressed this simple fact several times throughout this book, and I have done this on purpose, to make you really think about it and hopefully understand what it means. Smells simply do not exist to us!

This simple fact creates a huge difference between congenital and acquired anosmics. We are separated by an abyss. A person who loses her sense of smell knows, from own experience that smells exist, even if she cannot sense them anymore. She understands about good and bad smells, about things that smell and those that do not. Being born anosmic, I live in a world that is completely devoid of all smells. With your help I can learn rules for everyday life that help me fit in to your smell-crazy world, but *I can never really understand smells, because smells have never existed in my world.*

But in spite of this difference we all, both congenital and acquired anosmics, belong to the same community and there are several things that we share.

PART THREE

The anosmic world

ACQUIRED OR CONGENITAL

SO FAR I have mostly talked about anosmia without stressing the difference between the two major types of anosmia: acquired and congenital. There are similarities but in some ways they affect people differently.

"Acquired anosmia" means that a person had a functioning sense of smell since birth, but that something suddenly caused a loss of it. Food suddenly has little or no taste, she cannot sense changes in the weather or the shift of seasons through smells, she cannot smell flowers, her partner, her children, and so on. Not having to smell really bad odors does not compensate for the loss. A whole dimension of her world has suddenly disappeared.

For most of those afflicted it is only temporary. It only lasts a few days, some weeks, a few months, or at the worst a year or more, but they eventually get it back. But for some, time goes on and nothing changes. The loss seems to be permanent, and usually no one can tell them if or when they will get their sense of smell back. Many medical professionals have never heard of anosmia and have no knowledge about it. The lack of information and uncertainty of whether the sense of smell will come back or not is often described like a trauma. Those afflicted really lack and miss the ability to sense smells because it has suddenly changed their lives dramatically. It may lead to depression and sometimes even suicide. People who lose their sense of smell usually know exactly when it happened, and how long they have lived without it. If you ask them, they will tell you of all their visits to doctors and hospitals, of their despair of not getting any recommendations of treatments, or estimates of when it will return. Many of them spend a lot of time trying to find a cure on their own. Acquiring anosmia is usually a very traumatic experience.

Being congenital is quite different. To me it is not a question of not being able to sense smells. There are simply no smells in the world I experience and because of this I do not miss them. I live in a different world than people who can smell. In some ways my world is radically different from theirs, but I am so used to living in my world without smells that I seldom think about how different it is.

Researchers believe that about 20% of the population, that is every fifth (!) human, acquires temporary anosmia at some time during their lives. The majority regains it, but for about one percent of those afflicted, one in 500, it becomes permanent. They never get their sense of smell back. Acquired anosmia is thus fairly common.

For congenital anosmia the numbers are unreliable because most of us never visit a doctor or hospital to get it checked. Some researchers have tried to guess the prevalence of congenital anosmia based on available data, but the guesses vary between one in a thousand to one in a million births. So maybe a German study published in 2012 was right, when they concluded that somewhere between one and two in ten thousand are born with anosmia.

That congenital anosmia is unusual can also be shown indirectly. Almost everyone that joins the Facebook group *Congenital anosmia* says that it is the first time that they have gotten in touch with other anosmics. Being congenitally anosmic is so unusual that most anosmics live all their lives without ever meeting anyone else with the condition face-to-face. But then again, how would I know if I met another anosmic? It is a hidden disability and we almost never talk about it, so even if there were other anosmics around me, how would I know?

But how do you become anosmic?

What causes anosmia?

TO UNDERSTAND HOW people become anosmic requires some basic knowledge about the sense of smell. About the components of the olfactory system and how they function together.

Almost everything in our world emits smell molecules. Different substances emit different molecules. When the molecules enter the nose of a human being they react with smell receptors sitting in the mucous membranes in the upper part of the nose. The total area covered with smell receptors is about 5 cm^2 (roughly 0.8 in^2), which holds a total of about 50 million smell receptors, which can be divided into about 350 different kinds. This may sound like a large number, but for some dog breeds the area covered with receptor cells is about 15 times larger, so it is no wonder that dogs have a more sophisticated sense of smell than humans.

From the receptor cells, signals are sent through nerve fibers going up through the bone structure separating the nose cavity from the brain, up to the olfactory bulb which relays the signals into the smell center in the brain, that sits right above the olfactory bulb. By combining and interpreting the signals, a human can identify at least 10,000 different individual smells. Some researchers claim that the number should be much larger, that it could be as much as one million different smells. Irrespective of which number is correct, most smells are perceived as unpleasant. Maybe this tells us something about the original purpose of the olfactory system for humans: to identify and avoid things that are dangerous or unhealthy for us.

So what happens when someone becomes anosmic?

Acquired anosmia is usually caused by some kind of disease or physical damage. The list of diseases that can cause anosmia is very long and contain several fairly common diseases, like ordinary colds, sinusitis, polyps, diabetes, asthma, allergies, and so on. The direct cause of the anosmia is often that the disease induces inflammation in the areas where the olfactory receptor cells are situated. The inflammation prevents the smell receptors from detecting the smell molecules. If the inflammation is cured, the sense of smell usually starts functioning again, but sometimes a part of or the whole area with receptor cells has been damaged and then the anosmia may become permanent.

Also more uncommon diseases can distort or destroy the sense of smell. Among them are diseases connected to aging, like stroke, Alzheimer's and Parkinson's disease. To some extent, anosmia can actually be used as part of the diagnosis for these diseases. Kallmann's syndrome, a genetic disturbance of the sexual development, also belongs to this group. Anosmia can also appear together with multiple sclerosis (MS) and Cushing's syndrome. Medicines can also affect the sense of smell as a side effect, as does smoking.

Other causes of acquired anosmia are related to physical trauma. A hard blow on the head can damage the part of the brain that contains the smell center, or it could sever the nerves going up through the bone tissue from the receptor cells to the olfactory bulb. However, in many instances it is impossible to explain exactly what has happened and exactly why a person lost her sense of smell.

For congenital anosmia, on the other hand, some kind of

What causes anosmia?

genetic error is probably the most common cause. When the sense of smell is developing during fetal development, an error in the genetic code results in some kind of fault. Sometimes this is hereditary while at other times anosmia appears spontaneously. A medical examination can sometimes reveal that the anosmic lacks smell receptors in the nose, or that the nerves that should be going up through the bone structure are missing, or that the olfactory bulb is missing or underdeveloped, and so on.

Sometimes all parts are present, but there are no signals going from the smell receptor in the nose up to the brain. Sometimes something was damaged during birth, or fairly soon after birth. In these cases it is actually a kind of acquired anosmia, but the damage occurs so early in the child's life that she has no memory of being able to smell. Therefore, it will be experienced and described as congenital anosmia. Many times no explanation can be found, so the only thing to do is to accept that the person cannot sense smell and has no recollection of doing it.

What caused my anosmia? I do not know and it does not matter. This is a part of who I am, in the same way that my eyes are blue or that I have a good ear for music. This disinterest in the cause is a feeling I share with many congenital anosmics. But it is in strong contrast to the opinion of most acquired anosmics. They usually want to know very precisely what happened.

So what does the future hold for us? Are there any cures for anosmia?

ARE THERE CURES OR AIDS?

IF YOU ARE anosmic, are there any medical tricks to kick-start the olfactory system? The short answer is "No," but it depends on what the cause is.

If the anosmia is caused by inflammation inside the nose, treating it with anti-inflammatory medicine like antibiotics or cortisone can sometimes reduce the inflammation. If the inflammation is cured or at least reduced, the patient often regains her sense of smell. In some cases steroids have been successfully used as an alternative treatment to reduce the swelling.

If the anosmia is a result of brain damage, caused by a blow to the head from a hit or a fall, there is usually nothing anyone can do. In those cases the anosmia usually is permanent. But if the head trauma only severed the nerves going through the bone structure from the receptor cells in the nose up to the olfactory bulb, they can sometimes re-connect. Researchers are trying to find techniques to help this process. One such technique is to let people with acquired anosmia train with different smells. The patients are given a few distinct smells they are familiar with and try to smell these twice a day for several weeks or even months. In some cases such smell training may improve the sense of smell.

For congenital anosmia the situation is quite different. In many cases the cause is unknown, and without a cause it is impossible to know what to treat. When there is a clear cause for the anosmia, the most common appears to be a missing or not fully developed olfactory bulb, which cannot be treated, at least not with the current level of medical knowledge. In the future it may be possible, under certain conditions.

During the last few years some progress has been made in laboratory tests with mice. One of the techniques tested is gene therapy. It has been used to cause olfactory receptor cells to start developing and to grow new nerves to replace damaged ones in the nose of mice. This is very new research that so far has remained restricted to experiments in laboratories. Even if this technique should turn out to be successful in the long run, there is still a long way to go from experiments on mice to practical use on humans. Besides, it is still an open question how complete such a sense of smell would be. Would it really do any good?

However, there is another possible path, a line of development which could prove to be very useful, at least to us congenital anosmics: electronic noses.

Already sensors exist that can identify alcohol and smells coming from certain explosives, and more is coming. Several companies are developing other kinds of sensors for more normal conditions. The sensors come in two categories: passive and active.

One kind of passive sensor consists of a gel which reacts to certain substances or a specific kind of molecule and then changes color. That kind of sensor could be used in a household to inform an anosmic that it is time to ventilate the house, apartment or room, to prevent it from having a bad odor. There are other kinds of sensors which could be incorporated in clothes, to tell us if a shirt or sweater smelled of sweat.

The active products are meant to work like an electronic nose. You point the e-nose at something, it "sniffs" with a little built-in

Are there cures or aids?

fan, and then presents what it senses on a scale. In its simplest form it can recognize smells which tell if food is okay to eat or not. Such devices are already available, including a similar kind of sensor warning for gas leaking from gas stoves. A more advanced version could, possibly, both identify different smells and present the strength on a scale. There are also ideas about sensors that could be built into refrigerators and which would automatically warn when food in the refrigerator is beginning to smell badly.

Some products are already available, and companies say more will be available in a few years' time. Until then we will have to get along with the help of human noses. And in return we can actually help them sometimes. When I tell people that I am anosmic most of them realize that this means that I am not bothered by things that stink. Because of this my anosmia sometimes makes me a kind of superhero!

Anosmic superheros

IN OUR FAMILY I have always been the one to handle stinking things. When our children were sick, I sat with them when they were vomiting or having diarrhea, and took care of the filthy bed linen because, obviously, I was not bothered by the bad smells.

In our summer cottage we have an ecological toilet in which the poop ends up in a plastic bag in a kind of bucket. When full, you remove it and store it to produce mulch. Everyone else in the family has always detested doing this, so it has always been my job to take care of that.

If we have forgotten food in the refrigerator, it is usually my job to get rid of it. If it is food stored in glass jars I throw out the content and bring the jar to the recycling station. This is always my job. The others in my family usually avoid being in the kitchen until I have dumped the garbage in the dust bin.

But sometimes it gets really weird. We recently renovated a combined bathroom in our house. During the process three waste-pipes had to be opened and the stink traps removed. The plumber plugged the open waste-pipes with plastic bags to prevent the sewer stench from entering the house. Unfortunately one of the plugs was not airtight so the house slowly began to reek of sewer. Nobody wanted to enter the stinking bathroom, but to me the toilet was as smell-free as before, so it became my job to plug the leaking waste-pipe. No problem! Except for one little detail. Obviously, I had no idea which one of the three waste-pipes that was leaking. So I re-plugged all three anew, and hoped I got it right so the stench stopped seeping into the house.

Sometimes anosmia can have unexpected consequences. An anosmic working in a shop told about one occasion when a scruffy looking man entered the shop. He needed something special, so she helped him. It took about half an hour to find what he was looking for. When he had paid and left the shop her colleagues suddenly appeared and commended her for enduring him for half an hour in spite of the stench. What stench, she thought, and realized that her anosmia had made her treat him like any customer, instead of trying to get rid of him because of his odor. Maybe that was the reason for his being so extremely grateful when he left the store, thanking her so dearly. And maybe he was an anosmic, like her?

Anosmia can also be the cause of unintentional comedy. In high school we dissected frogs during a biology lab, and everyone was complaining loudly about how disgusting it was, except me. I did not understand how a dead frog could be so disgusting. Recently an acquired anosmic told a similar story, but with a small addition. The reason she did not find it disgusting was because she did not smell the formalin which the frogs were stored in. Formalin apparently smells awful and reading her story I suddenly realized that maybe I had misunderstood the situation during all these years? Maybe it was the smell of formalin my classmates were complaining about all those years ago, and not the frogs?

A female anosmic told a story about when she began dating the man who later was to be her husband. He was an ice hockey player. She had told him from the start that she was anosmic, but he just shrugged and said "Okay," and probably did not understand what it really meant. The first time she followed him to a game, she went down to the locker room after the game and gave him a hug and a kiss while he was still in his gear. He froze, looked at her and exclaimed, "Wow! You really don't smell me! I have never before met a girl who wants to hug after a game". She later learned that after a game the equipment used by the players smells really bad, but of course not to her.

One occasion my anosmia was an advantage to me was during my military service. We were training how to protect ourselves against chemical weapons. We had to walk around all day in rainwear and a gas-mask. Everyone was complaining about how awful the rubber masks were and how awful the air felt when they breathed through the filter in the masks. As far as I remember I thought wearing the mask was quite okay. The air I breathed felt like all air always does. It reminded me of the scuba mask I used for diving during the summers.

At the end of the day our commanding officer told us we were to move to a cleaning station where everyone could remove their masks and the exercise would end. That was, everyone except two voluntary guards who would remain in full gear until the exercise was finished. Any volunteers? I stepped forward, of course, because I did not mind wearing the gas-mask a little longer. It even kept my face warm in the chilly autumn afternoon. The others just laughed and shook their heads, so the officer had to appoint one more volunteer. We moved to the cleaning station, where everyone except us two guards had to strip, wash themselves outdoors, with cold water, in 5 degrees centigrade (F 41). They swore and asked angrily if I had known about this? I shook my head and smiled inside my mask, fully dressed and warm.

When I look back I remember the others were complaining about the smell from the rubber masks, but when this took place it never occurred to me that I experienced the gas-mask differently than they did. I do remember that I did not understand why everyone else thought the masks were so awful to wear, but I never made the connection with my anosmia. And here we have another difference between my world and the smelling world. I never experience things disgusting or nauseating in the way that others do.

Nothing is disgusting

WHEN TALKING ABOUT bad smells there is one very interesting detail: feelings of disgust. If you can smell, some smells can cause physical reactions. The smell of vomit, feces, rotten food, etcetera, is so disgusting that it may cause nausea or even vomiting. The biological function of this is to warn us and make us avoid unhealthy places or bad food.

Is there anything similar for an anosmic? No, there is not. It is rather the other way around. Someone who knows how feces and vomit smells associates the sight of such things with feelings of disgust. So just seeing something like that, without smelling it, can cause nausea. For some it is enough to hear someone talking about something that stinks, to get a reaction. If this happens during a dinner, the person might lose her appetite and stop eating. Never having smelled any bad stuff I have never done that association or connection, so stinking things like vomit and feces are not disgusting to me in the way they are to those who can smell.

The following story which I got from an anosmic woman, describes it beautifully.

She was going home by subway during rush hours. It was crowded on the platform when the train arrived. It stopped, the doors opened, and suddenly the crowd disappeared in front of her. Everyone moved towards the adjacent wagons although the one in front of her was empty. She did not understand what was happening and entered anyway. When she walked towards the empty wagon, she looked around and saw how people looked at her, talked with each other and pointed towards her, while they were trying to get aboard the crowded adjacent wagons. She entered the empty wagon, looked around, and saw something on the floor in the middle of the aisle. It looked like poop. She smiled and sat down, and enjoyed having a whole wagon all by herself.

For someone who knows how it smelled in the wagon, the prospect of sitting there would probably be completely out of the question. For the anosmic woman the wagon was smell free, so why not enjoy a wagon that is all yours? I would probably have done the same thing.

Another similar story:

An anosmic student came to a lecture early, so the room was empty when she entered. She sat down at one of the front rows and put her feet up on the backrest in front of her. After a while another student entered, made a face and went out again. More students arrived, and they all did the same. Finally it was crowded outside the lecture room, but she was alone inside. The teacher entered, also making a face, and told her that she had probably stepped in dog poo or something similar just before entering the lecture room. She was asked to clean her shoes and the lecture was moved to another room while they ventilated the first one.

There is probably no difference in the way anosmics and others experience things like spiders, slithering worms, centipedes or cockroaches, because then it is the sight and not the smell that triggers a possibly unpleasant feeling. But if I see something I find disgusting, all I have to do is close my eyes or look in another direction, and the problem is solved. If someone who can smell experiences disgusting smells she cannot smell in another direction, because the smell is all around her, and nor can she close her nose. Even if she did hold her nose, she would eventually have to breath and the smells would return. The only solution would be to leave the place that smells or avoid going there in the first place, like shown by the stories above.

However, although I am never bothered by disgusting smells, there is a complicating detail. I have been told that unpleasant smells can impregnate one's clothes, hair and even skin. As a result I could carry the unpleasant smells with me after having been in a place with a bad smell, without knowing it.

But smells have another, less obvious effect. They affect how people perceive the world around them in a more general sense.

Cleaner but less beautiful

PEOPLE ASSESS MUCH of their surroundings based on smells. I do not, of course. Just as I cannot sense bad smells I cannot sense pleasant smells. In my description of an ordinary day in the beginning of this book I mention not sensing the smell of spring flowers or the wet grass which I, obviously, never do.

When I scrub the floor, I can see that it is wet, and I can see if possible stains disappeared, but when the floor has dried, there is nothing to remind me that it has just been scrubbed. If my wife enters the room she immediately comments about the pleasant scent of soap and the room feeling clean. If she brings flowers from the garden, she praise their fragrance. I see the flowers, how they differ in shape and color, but that is all.

It is of course the same with everything that smells nice. Pleasant aromas add something to the experience when people perceive beautiful things or the world around them. The scents make the world slightly more beautiful. My world consequently is a bit less beautiful, maybe you could even say that it is a bit uglier than the world that others live in.

But the biggest difference is probably the opposite.

Sometimes when we come home from work, my wife remarks about the air indoors being stale, or about a bad smell coming from the garbage we forgot to take outside in the morning. Towels can smell bad, and bed linen, the cats' litter box, sweaty clothes, and so on. There are apparently a lot of things around us that can smell bad to a person with a functioning sense of smell.

We have horses. When we get home after having groomed them and taken a ride around the village where we live, my wife sometimes says that our riding gear is reeking of horse smells. But to me they feel exactly the same as before we went down to the stables. Just as I cannot sense nice smells, I cannot sense bad smells, no matter how strong they are.

All this means that I could be somewhere where it is reeking of dirt, feces, mold, or something else that is unhealthy, without knowing it. As a result, I always perceive the world as cleaner than it actually is, and this is probably the biggest difference between my world and the one perceived by someone who can smell.

My world is essentially clean.

Of course there may be litter on the floor, clothes may have visible stains, I can see that the trash bag in the kitchen is full, or that someone forgot to flush the toilet. But apart from what I see, there is nothing more. If I look away there is nothing to remind me of the dirt and even if I see it, it does not evoke emotions of disgust or nausea. This creates a big divider between the smelling world that others experience and my smell-free world: My world is always clean, and theirs is always a bit dirty.

This affects not only how I perceive my surroundings, but also people I meet. To me everyone is clean, in the sense that in my world no one ever smells of sweat or dirt.

Beyond making the world cleaner or a bit less beautiful or uglier, smells can also create a kind of context, a feeling of really being enveloped in your surroundings.

When I and my wife walk in a forest we see trees, plants, rocks, and we hear birds, possibly insects, the wind, and so on. But on top of that, my wife will also be surrounded by the smells of the forest. The smells will amplify the sensation of being in exactly that kind of forest, and will thereby also amplify the perception of the surrounding space. If she closes her eyes, she can still sense the forest around her. When I close my eyes, the sounds remain, nothing else. In a way the forest disappears when it is no longer visible.

This relation between smells and the surrounding space can also create an illusion of crowdedness, that the surroundings are filled with something. A conference room with lots of people, a store filled with customers, a restaurant, the subway, etc. They can all feel crowded, filled up, having bad air, making it unpleasant or oppressive to breathe in there. To me the air is usually the same everywhere, so I do not experience the same feeling of crowdedness. To a person who can smell, smells can thus strengthen the way a place is perceived.

Another difference has to do with which of our senses defines our horizon of perception. For an anosmic like me this horizon is limited by what I can see and hear. Because smells can travel and swiftly be diffused in a completely different way than light and sound, and over long distances, others can sense smells that originated far beyond sight or hearing distance. Being anosmic I, therefore, have a more limited horizon of perception.

If I am sitting in a room, I can see the room and perhaps hear what happens in adjacent rooms. A person sensing smells can get information about what happens in other rooms, like telling the person that someone is preparing dinner or making coffee in the kitchen. I do not get any such information from my surroundings. It comes as a surprise to me when someone suddenly says, "Coffee is ready".

It is the same outdoors. Someone visiting a new city might suddenly sense a smell coming from the street corner, alerting her to what is around the corner. When she reaches the corner her sight can confirm the forewarning her sense of smell gave her. I have no idea what is hidden behind the street corner until I turn the corner and can see what is there. It is the same when in the countryside. The sense of smell can tell you that a farmer is fertilizing his fields with manure long before you see the field or hear the tractor. A smell of salt water and seaweed can reveal there is a sea beyond the forest, several kilometers away. To me it will come as a complete surprise to see the farmer driving the tractor across the field, and I might not even be able to see from a distance that he is spreading manure. In the same way it will come as a surprise that there is a sea where the forest ends.

My horizon of perception is always a little closer than it is if you can smell. One might thus say that the world I perceive is smaller than the world you perceive with a fully functioning sense of smell. But smells do not only affect how we perceive what we experience. Smells also connect to memories.

MEMORIES AND TIME

SMELLS ARE VERY closely connected to memories. They have the ability to make people remember specific moments and situations from the past, especially from their childhood. What is interesting is that such memories usually appear unexpectedly, and they are usually related to events that the person has forgotten. They are therefore referred to as "involuntary" memories, because they cannot be consciously recalled. Typical examples are when someone smells food that was served during childhood, or a detergent that was used where she grew up. It can also be a specific combination of smells. Often it is happy memories, but not always. Smells may also provoke memories of unpleasant or sad occasions that the person has repressed. This way the sense of smell can unexpectedly and uncontrollably evoke forgotten or repressed memories from the past.

A congenital anosmic of course has no such system, nor anything that replaces it. So I don't risk being unexpectedly reminded of my past. However, several of the anosmics I have been in touch with have told me that music can evoke memories in a way that at least partially remind of the involuntary memories evoked by smells. I have experienced the same thing myself, but they usually are rather blurred memories. Certain music by The Beatles usually reminds me of playing with some specific toys I had as a child. Probably because my older brother kept playing that music over and over at the time I used those toys. Other music can remind me of reading a specific book, probably for the same reason. But most of the time music only reminds me of being in a certain mood, not really reminding me of a certain environment or event.

The ability of smells to evoke memories can be seen as a way to affect the perception of time backwards. But because smells can often be transported far beyond what one can see, smells can also affect what is happening right now, by giving a forewarning about things that will happen, later on.

When someone is cooking dinner, the smells are spreading throughout the house, and those who can smell are forewarned that dinner time is approaching. Smells can stimulate the appetite and thus bring a kind of joy even before the dinner is ready. During the dinner the smells affect the perceived flavor of the food, and when the dinner is finished, the smells may remain for quite a while, reminding everyone of the finished meal. This way the smells extend the temporal horizon of the meal. If someone is baking a cake, the home will smell of the newly baked cake for several hours, and give a premonition of the coming joy when the cake will be eaten.

Smells can prolong the temporal horizon backwards, but also prolong it forward in time, by giving a hint of something that is to come.

If one adds the wider horizon, the increased sense of presence, and the wider temporal horizon that smells can create, the result is a world that is made larger thanks to smells. Being anosmic one ends up with the opposite. My world is limited to what I can see and hear, and it is thus smaller than the world experienced by those who can smell.

I never get any forewarning that someone is preparing dinner, and when the dinner is finished, it is really finished. To me there is nothing lingering to remind me of the dinner. When the cake is put aside, nothing reminds me that someone has baked a cake, or that the cake is there to be eaten later. I cannot see what is waiting around the corner, or see what was there earlier but is no longer present. I cannot sense what is beyond what I can see and hear. I can only experience what is present, here and now, and I experience it instantly when I look around. Maybe this makes me more aware of the present?

Because of my anosmia I do not experience the extra dimension that the smell can give you when you see a beautiful flower. But it also means that I live in a world devoid of stench and foul odors. Put together this means that being anosmic, I experience a world that is slightly smaller, not quite as beautiful but much cleaner than the world of people who can smell. Does this difference make me disabled?

Am I disabled?

IS ANOSMIA A disability? A handicap? This question is frequently discussed in the Facebook group "Congenital anosmia," and members express opposite opinions. Some claim that they do not suffer from the anosmia, that it does not affect their day-to-day life, and that they are not restricted by their anosmia. On top of that, there are people who have more severe problems, so consequently congenital anosmia is not a disability. Others claim, with equal strength, that anosmia is of course a disability. We lack one of the five senses!

In Sweden there is an official distinction between a disability that is only a reduction in an ability and a disability that is a hindrance in day-to-day life. Anosmia is without question a disability in the former sense, but is it a hindrance? I lack one of the five senses that people usually have, but has it really affected my life in any way? Is it really a hindrance? My answer is without doubt "Yes!" To me it is obvious that anosmia is not only a disability in a formal way, but it very much affects my everyday life.

You might think that the biggest problem would be to identify bad food, but it is not. The toughest part is hygiene. This is at the same time the one thing that has the largest impact on how we are judged by others. However, it is not so much about hygiene itself as it is about social conventions.

A lot of the interactions between people in our modern

society are connected to smells. You are supposed to be "neat and clean," meaning that neither you nor the clothes you are wearing should smell of sweat or dirt. It is a part of good manners to smell nicely. Clothes are supposed to smell from being washed in washing powder scented with perfumes. You are expected to smell nice from using scented soap, shampoo and deodorant. Toothpaste and mouthwash should be used to prevent bad breath. We are constantly exposed to commercials for all sorts of products that together with regular showers, washing your hair, brushing your teeth, and changing your clothes, should guarantee that we always smell nice.

A person who does not follow these unwritten rules, who walks around spreading an unpleasant smell, is seen as a bit odd, weird, eccentric, or outright unpleasant. To be cut off from all of this, and not even knowing what smells are, sometimes results in one not being able to participate in or even understand what others are experiencing. If I do not know if I or my clothes smell, how can I know to what degree I live up to the smelling standards set by the rest of the society? The simple answer is that I cannot. This is and has always been the big problem with my anosmia.

And on top of having to remember all the unwritten rules, there are all those comments about smells that are always flying about, passing me without really connecting, ever since I was a child. Resulting in an undefined and elusive feeling of being left outside, not really being a part of the conversation, not really understanding, only pretending to do so.

Writing this book has been a real eye-opener to me. I never really thought that my anosmia affected my life. Looking back and really thinking about it, I realize that it has always been there, in the back of my mind, worrying me. But not knowing anything about it, not knowing how to handle it, and not having anyone to guide me, I have simply tried not to worry about it and to improvise some rules of my own about hygiene and clothes and such things.

Looking back at my childhood and teenage years, I realize that there were times when I probably did not handle it very well. My parents did not know that I was anosmic until I was in my teens, and even after being told about it they did not understand what it really meant and how it affected me. And I myself, of course, did not understand at all. When my mind was occupied with something else, I simply forgot the few smell rules I had invented. My parents did remind me, and made sure I remembered to shower and change clothes, to keep me "neat and clean". However, initially not knowing about my anosmia and later on not remembering or understanding it, there was no systematic control or training. And when I moved out and went to university, there was no one around to help me and remind me.

What I have also realized, looking back, was that the only person who has really taught me about smells, how to think about daily routines, and how to stay "neat and clean," has been my wife. But because neither she nor I have really understood what my anosmia means, and how it affects me, there has never been any systematic training. Instead she has made remarks over the years when I missed something, when I have forgotten to take a shower, forgotten to change clothes, and so on. She has also been forced to carry the responsibility to keep our home clean, and tell me when things needed to be cleaned so I could take my part of the work. Her remarks and comments have often felt irritating, or even unfair, but without them I would never have learned how to behave in accordance with the unwritten smell rules of our society. So I guess I owe it to her that I have been able to act in a socially acceptable way over the years.

Looking back I cannot help wondering how I functioned

before meeting her, and how we could end up being married and having a family. There are scientific studies showing that anosmics have more problems finding a partner, have fewer relationships, and feel more insecure in their current relationships. Maybe I was simply lucky?

My anosmia has forced me to consciously handle and actively think about something that is totally irrelevant to me, and which I cannot even understand: how others perceive that things smell. How this has affected me I am finally slowly beginning to understand. But what is really unfair about it is that I will have to go on like this for the rest of my life. There will never come a day when I can say "That's it! I am done, and can forget about smells from now on".

And then there is the problem with food, which I described in an earlier chapter. My inability to judge whether the food is okay to eat or not. A disability which has sent anosmics around the world to hospitals after having eaten food that was spoiled and therefore unhealthy to eat, which has caused me to drink milk that has gone sour, eat bread with mold, and so on.

So yes, congenital anosmia is a disability that constantly affects my day-to-day life, even when I do not think about it.

And still, how come I do not miss my missing sense of smell?

NOT MISSING WHAT YOU MISS

TO MISS SOMETHING can mean that something is absent and using that definition I miss a sense of smell. But I do not miss it in the sense that I yearn for it, or feel a loss. The thing is you can only yearn for something that you have had, or at least have some conception of what it is.

A person who is congenitally blind cannot understand what it means to see, and cannot understand what light and darkness is. Analogous to this, being a congenital anosmic I cannot really understand what it is to sense smells, or what the difference is between different smells. I have no personal experience of what smells are. All I know is what others have told me. To me smells are only words, something I read about in books and magazines, and hear others talk about. But to me they do not really exist. That is why it is impossible for me to understand this thing "smell," and to understand a world with smells.

A person with functioning eyesight who is blindfolded gets a glimpse of what it would be like to become blind, but not how it is to be congenitally blind. For a person who has sensed smells all her life, it is equally impossible to understand what it is really like to be congenitally anosmic, to never have experienced smells and therefor not know what they are.

You may know that we are surrounded by magnetic fields. The earth's magnetic field is so strong that we can easily get a simple reading of it using an ordinary compass. But that's not all.

Every electronic appliance we have in our homes, and all electric cables around us, also create magnetic fields. This means that all rooms in a building contain several magnetic fields, with different strengths and directions, all mixed up.

Imagine that you travel to some far away place. While being there you sometimes hear people comment on something that you do not quite understand. The people living in this far away place seems to sense something which you do not. After a while you realize that people around you actually can sense the shape, strength and direction of magnetic fields when they enter a room or move about in nature. In school you were taught that there is such a thing as magnetic fields, but you would not have any experience of what it feels like to sense them yourself, with your own "magnetic field sense". You would be "magnetic field"-blind.

That is exactly what it is like to be congenitally anosmic. I only know of smells as an abstraction, something I have heard others talk about, read about in books, like magnetic fields and other abstract knowledge. That is why I, being a congenital anosmic, do not miss my sense of smell, although it is missing.

But even if I do not mind being anosmic, I still have questions and want to learn more about it. So where can I find answers?

THE ANOSMIC COMMUNITY

ONE OF THE problems with having an unknown and uncommon condition is that you have no one to talk to. As far as I know there is no congenital anosmic in my vicinity, so I have no one with whom I can discuss and share my thoughts about anosmia. Of course I can talk to my family, friends and colleagues but they can all smell and do not really understand. Talking to people who can smell about anosmia usually becomes a kind of one-way dissemination of information because they know and understand very little. What you really need is to talk to other anosmics. One obvious connection point is Facebook.

There are several small groups out there, usually only having a few members, but there are also two quite large groups: "Anosmics of the World, Unite!" and "Congenital anosmia".

The first one, *Anosmics of the World, Unite!*, is a wide and general group, open to everyone interested in some kind of anosmia. In the spring of 2017 it had about 1600 members and it is a very active group, constantly growing.

Because acquired anosmia is much more common than congenital anosmia, the group is dominated by acquired anosmics. As a result most of the discussions in this group are about how people lost their sense of smell, about all they miss, about possible cures and information from meetings with the medical profession. The posts in there can be divided in two main groups: Support and information.

Lars Lundqvist

Losing a sense is always traumatic but losing a sense and then not getting proper attention and information from the medical profession makes things even worse. There are no support groups, no psychologists trained in handling patients with acute anosmia, not even relevant information for those stricken. The Facebook group is for many anosmics their only support group, their only option if they want to talk to people who understand their situation. I think the group has a very important mission in this respect.

The information part is probably just as important. A person who lost her sense of smell needs practical advice about how to handle things in day-to-day life. There is a need for information about food, possible cures, and so on.

One of the advantages of having a large group with many active members is that no matter what kind of questions people post, there is almost always someone else who has relevant experiences to share. Because of this the group automatically emphasizes the feeling of not being alone.

Sometimes the discussions become a bit heated. Usually as a result of differences in opinions or experiences between congenital and acquired anosmics. Although there are similarities between congenital and acquired anosmia, there is one crucial aspect where there are no similarities at all. A person who was born with a sense of smell knows what smells are and how it feels to be able to smell. Even if she later loses the sense and becomes anosmic she still knows what it is to smell and understand the concept of smelling. Having once experienced the smelling world she cannot really understand the totally smell-free world of congenital anosmics. And being congenitally anosmic it is impossible to truly understand the utter despair some acquired anosmics express when they talk about their loss. Although I intellectually understand their reaction, my own emotional reaction is sometimes "What's the big fuss? You lost something that doesn't exist." But although that may sometimes be my gut reaction, decency requires that we all accept the emotions and experiences of others.

Trying to understand people who have lost their sense of smell has given me a unique glimpse into the world of smells, showing me what I cannot experience myself from a different angle. And for all those anosmics who were born with a sense of smell, this Facebook group is a gold mine of information and support so I can really recommend it to other anosmics.

The second group is called *Congenital anosmia* and, as the name suggest, it primarily targets people who were born without a sense of smell. In the spring of 2017 it had about 1300 members. They literally come from all over the world and are of all ages. The majority of members in the group are congenital anosmics, but there are other members as well, e.g. parents of children with anosmia. The discussions deal with subjects like how daily life is affected by anosmia, about reactions from family and friends, how different foods taste and how we experience the world, but we also share jokes. An interesting detail is that although we have all lived with this our whole lives, most new members know very little about anosmia and the discussions are often eye openers.

A recurring event in the group is the reaction from new members. The most common opening line from new members is that this is the first time they have come in touch with other congenital anosmics. It was the same for me. I can still remember the feeling when I was admitted to the group. It was a combination of relief, joy and surprise. I had lived for so many years being alone with my anosmia, never really thinking about it, probably in a way suppressing it. And then suddenly I found people who were exactly like me. Who immediately understood when I asked or described something. Yes! Awesome! Finally!

Lars Lundqvist

One of the big differences between being born anosmic and losing your sense of smell as an adult is that being congenitally anosmic you are totally cut off from one aspect of the world everyone else experiences. You have no perception at all about 'smell' but growing up in an environment where everyone else can smell, you mimic people around you and learn to behave like them. So without being aware of it you actually learn to behave as if you can smell. But what is very obvious from the discussions in the group is that because we have had to do this on our own, without the help from people around us, we have all adopted slightly different strategies to cope with our anosmia.

I recommend this group to everyone who has congenital anosmia and I hope that the group will continue to grow.

There are also other communities out there. The Yahoo group "Anosmia" describes itself as "mailing list and resources for people lacking the sense of smell". Most discussions are about acquired anosmia and it is the same with the Reddit group "Anosmia". On Twitter a search for "anosmia" results in several users and tweets but at the time of writing this book, most of them were not very active or recent.

One of the few active organizations focusing on smell and taste disorders is FifthSense (www.fifthsense.org.uk). It is a non-profit charity organization based in the UK, established in 2012. Its vision is "for the senses of smell and taste to be recognized as being essential to our lives, health and general wellbeing," and it aims at educating society as well as providing support and advice for people with smell and taste disorders.

There is a lot of good information at their web site. Information about taste and smell disorders, ongoing research, advice on how to cope with day-to-day problems, and so on. They organize workshops, attend at various public events, and try to spread information to both society in general and to the medical profession.

Most information deals with problems with or loss of the sense of smell, so most of the information about anosmia is about acquired anosmia. However, there is a special page on congenital anosmia (www.fifthsense.org.uk/congenital-anosmia/), written by someone who understands our special situation.

Becoming a member is free and they accept members from all over the world.

There is also research going on in several places around the world. The Monell Center in Pennsylvania (www.monell.org) and the Center for Smell and Taste at the University of Florida (cst.ufl.edu), both in the USA, are two examples of research organisations that do quite a lot of research on anosmia, both acquired and congenital. They both have relevant information on their web sites, they both have researchers that follow what is happening in the anosmic Facebook groups and they sometimes want volunteers for their research. So it is well worth the time to check out their web sites from time to time.

Thanks to the Facebook groups and FifthSense I have been able to talk to other anosmics and learn a lot about what it really means to be anosmic. One of the aspects I would never have thought about without input from others is how being anosmic affects my ability to understand my own language.

ANOSMIA AND LANGUAGE

ONE CONSEQUENCE OF my inability to smell is that it prevents me from really understanding common words. There are numerous words describing bad smells, bad air and our surroundings: disgusting, nauseous, unsavory, dead, stale, musty, frowsty, whiffy, insipid, flavorless, vapid, spicy, confined, sweetish, sour, moldy, vomit, poop, urine, etcetera. Although I know what all these words mean, intellectually, I have no emotional connection to them, because they all relate to smells, which means I do not understand them. I guess you could compare with how a congenitally blind person would relate to the concept of colors. Obviously, the same goes for words that describe pleasant scents.

Maybe someone objects and thinks that surely I can understand that air can feel sweetish or sour? After all I do know the tastes sweet and sour. Yes, I know how sugar and vinegar taste, but I simply cannot translate that to the air I breath. I sometimes try to convince myself that I do understand how sour air should feel, but the truth is I do not. To me, air is never anything else than just air and it does not have a taste.

Languages are full of such descriptions of smells, and humans very often describe their surroundings with smells. We have horses and people knowing this sometimes say that the smell of their surroundings remind them of a stable, a farm, manure, urine, hay, ensilage, and so on. Outdoors it can smell like spring, summer, autumn or winter, descriptions that are completely incomprehensible to me because to me the air is the same all year round. Soap, detergents and fabric softeners are often marketed with words that describe places, like meadow or seashore. When I think of a meadow I think of insects buzzing, and seashore makes me think of sand. Neither of them are good associations for getting things clean. And soap can be called 'milk and honey'. How is something sweet and sticky supposed to make me think of getting clean hands?

Another aspect of language has to do with how anosmia is referred to by people who can smell. Because there is no simple, everyday name for anosmia, I have chosen to use the words 'anosmia' and 'anosmic' throughout this book. But sometimes when I read about anosmia the term 'nose blind' is used. That is a very bad term because it tends to lead ones thoughts in the wrong direction.

The word 'blind' is often used metaphorically to describe 'not being aware of' something. Being blind to something means not wanting to see, pretending not to see, ignore, not pay attention to, and so on. 'Nose blind' might thus imply that a person is 'blind to smells', that she actually knows what smells are, but for some reason cannot or chooses not to be able to sense them. That way 'nose blind' misses one of the key concepts of congenital anosmia: that congenital anosmics do not have any self perceived experience of smells and, therefore, do not know what smells are.

The second problem is that 'nose blind' is used for all kinds of problems related to the sense of smell, including a reduced ability to smell, being unable to sense specific smells, and also olfactory fatigue, meaning "the gradual acclimatization to the smells of one's home, car, or belongings, in which the affected does not notice them," and that is definitely not applicable to congenital anosmics.

Anosmia and language

So please, use the words "anosmic" and "anosmia" when you talk about not having a sense of smell.

With this we are approaching the end of this book. But two important questions remain to be answered.

Epilogue—Two final questions

IN THIS BOOK I have described how being anosmic has affected my life and the way I experience the world. Everyday problems, advantages and disadvantages, frustration and sorrow, but also happiness and comic situations. But two big questions remain to be answered.

The first question is: if someone offered me a treatment that would give me a fully functioning sense of smell, would I accept it?

A person who has lived most of her life being able to smell, but who suddenly lost that ability, would probably answer with a loud "Yes!" and start crying out of happiness for finally being cured. But I am not sure. I do not know if I would dare. And in a way I don't really see the point. Why would I want to get a sense that I never had and do not understand?

I read an interesting view on this on a blog written by a young female anosmic. How would she react if someone offered her a magical potion which would suddenly give her the ability to sense smells? Her guess was that she would accept the gift, but hide it somewhere safe, and only look at it from time to time but without using it. Just knowing that the possibility was there, within reach for her to use if she wanted to, would be enough to make her content with her current life. I sympathize with her line of thought.

People who can smell very often talk about this thing they call "smell," but I am not sure if it really exists. At least I have never experienced something like that. So why would I want to be subjected to a perhaps difficult treatment to get a new ability, a new sense which I would not know how to use or what it would feel like to have?

I think that when anosmics fantasize about being able to smell, it is not about regaining it, but to have never lived without it. If I suddenly got a sense of smell, how would it change my life if I could sense only some smells, not all? And what if my brain only learned to handle bad smells? Or what if all the millions of smell receptors started working at full speed all at once, and showered my brain with thousands of individual and unknown smells, how would I react? When you are an infant, your brain gradually learns to handle all the sensory input. But to have the smelling system suddenly activated when you are an adult would probably cause an extreme mental overload. I would have no references, nothing to compare it with and would not be able to identify the smells that were suddenly flooding my brain. I would probably move from a quiet, safe, smell-free clean environment, into a smelly, dirty, mental and sensory chaos.

The bottom line is that it is completely impossible for me to imagine what it would be like to have a sense of smell whether it was functioning perfectly or not. I have nothing to compare it with. So in spite of realizing that my anosmia is a disability which has affected my life in many ways, I think I would say, "No, thank you" if I got the offer. Still, thirty years ago I might have answered differently.

The second and final question is: would my life have been different if I had had a functioning sense of smell? My anosmia has without doubt affected my life, but has it restricted my life in any way? Has my anosmia made me refrain from something, or has it hindered me, in my professional career, socially, or in some other way?

This question is impossible to answer. I cannot know in what way my personal interests and hobbies, my social life, education, choice of career, professional relations, etcetera, were affected by being anosmic. I do not know if I would have been a different person had I had a functioning sense of smell since birth. All I know is that so far I have lived my whole life in a world where there are no smells, and that my world will remain without smells for the rest of my life. After all, that is the way the world is to me. Without smells.

I belong to the small minority in the world that are congenitally anosmic. This is usually described by others as an inability to sense smells, but that is not correct. In their world there might be smells, but in the world I experience there are none. My world lacks a dimension that exists in their world. It lacks some of the temptations connected to food and candy, and some of the disturbances caused by dirt and pollution. I do not risk being involuntarily reminded of things in my past or of places I once visited. I live here and now, and the only reality that exists to me is what I can see and hear. Therefore I experience a world that is smaller, maybe less beautiful but much cleaner than the world that others experience. Maybe that makes my world a bit meager in their eyes, but not to me.

This is the world I know, my world. A world without smells.

ACKNOWLEDGEMENT

THIS BOOK IS based not only on my own experiences but also on what I have learned from blogs, articles, scientific studies, and stories that other anosmics have told me. I thank the members of the Facebook group "Congenital Anosmia" for all their input and Jacqueline Kowalczyk for letting me borrow her story about the birthday cakes.

The parts dealing with how we perceive the world around us were inspired by thoughts and ideas presented by Marta Tafalla at the University of Barcelona, especially her article "A World Without the Olfactory Dimension" (2013, The Anatomical Record 296:1287–1296).

Finally, I thank Tom Elliot and Karin-Marijke Vis for editing my manuscript and encouraging me to publish it.

THANK YOU FOR READING THIS BOOK!

I HOPE YOU liked it.
If you have any questions, feel free to get in touch.
A short review where you bought the book would be hugely appreciated.
Sincerely, Lars Lundqvist
anosmia@icloud.com
congenitalanosmia.wordpress.com

www.ingramcontent.com/pod-product-compliance
Lightning Source LLC
Chambersburg PA
CBHW020519290526
45786CB00002B/667